EATING WITH
CONSCIENCE

D0059448

EATING WITH CONSCIENCE

The Bioethics of Food

Dr. Michael W. Fox

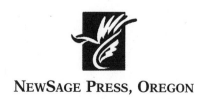

NewSage Press, Oregon

Eating with Conscience:
The Bioethics of Food

Copyright ©1997 Michael W. Fox
ISBN 0-939165-30-9

All rights reserved. No part of this book may be reproduced, transmitted, or used in any form without written permission from the publisher, except brief quotations embodied in literary articles and reviews.

The views in this book are those of the author and not necessarily that of the publisher or of any other individual or organization. The publisher assumes no responsibility for errors, inaccuracies, omissions, or any other inconsistency and cannot be held responsible for any loss or damages resulting from information contained within the book.

Address Inquiries to:
NewSage Press
PO Box 607
Troutdale, OR 97060-0607
503-695-2211; fax: 503-695-5406
Email: newsage@teleport.com
Web Site: http://www.teleport.com/~newsage

Book design by John Rodal
Production assistance by Nancy L. Doerrfeld-Smith

Illustrations in the book by Sue Coe, taken from her book *Dead Meat*, published by Four Walls Eight Windows, 1996.

Printed in the United States on recycled paper with soy ink.

Distributed in the United States and Canada by Publishers Group West
1-800-788-2123

Library of Congress Cataloging-in-Publication Data

Fox, Michael W. , 1937-
    Eating with conscience : the bioethics of food / Michael W. Fox.
      p. cm.
    Includes bibliographical references and index.
    ISBN 0-939165-30-9
    1. Agriculture--Moral and ethical aspects. 2. Bioethics.
  I. Title.
  BJ52.5.F69 1997
  179'.3--dc21   97-34714
                                               CIP

1 2 3 4 5 6 7 8 9 10

Acknowledgments

I owe much for the completion of this book to my wife and coworker, Deanna Krantz, and to my many professional and personal friends and colleagues. They have helped me in so many ways. This book is barely an adequate acknowledgment.

A special word of appreciation goes to my executive associate, Ms. Ellen Truong, who has put my words into manuscript form and into countless revisions. I am also grateful for the fine and professional editorial work of my publisher Maureen R. Michelson of NewSage Press, and copy editor, Tracy A. Smith. Countless hours have been spent to craft the bits and pieces of my original manuscript into a book, which is a clear call to everyone who eats—-and that includes you.

Contents

Chapter Nine

Change of Conscience: Actions and Solutions
> Initiatives for Concerned and Conscientious Consumers
> The Ten Commandments of Humane Organic
>> Sustainable Agriculture
> Chefs Join the Revolution
> Consumer Beware: Products from Animal Suffering
> Pets and Pet Food
> Gourmet Products to Avoid
> Community Supported Agriculture

Introduction

A Vision

Eating with Conscience is a call to consumers, farmers, and policy makers to establish a green alliance with each other. The slogan "Dirt First!" of the organic farming movement is worth reflection. Perhaps we need to speak of a brown rather than a green alliance. We need to repair the broken connections between the soil itself, the well-being of farmers, ranchers, consumers, and the humane treatment of farm animals and the environment. This book investigates why and how we broke these vital connections, and how we can—and must—restore them for the good of all.

This has been a difficult book for me to write. The enormity and complexity of the reality of how harmfully humans raise animals and grow crops for food is almost overwhelming. However, I am hopeful this book will move consumers, farmers, and policy makers to help revolutionize agriculture. My hope is for the industrial world to evolve into a sustainable rather than a self-destructive one. For this to happen we must continually educate ourselves and others, and accept personal responsibility for the changes necessary to preserve the natural world that still remains.

Dr. Michael W. Fox

Chapter One

Why Eat with Conscience?

*We do not find ourselves until
we see ourselves in the eyes of those
who are other than human.*

Loren Eiseley, anthropologist

We must begin the most important consumer revolution of the next millennium—transforming how our food is grown and what we choose to eat. The urgency of this revolution is undeniable, and the possibility for change lies within each one of us.

There is a quiet holocaust taking place worldwide in the animal kingdom and in the environment, which I call "agricide." Human beings are the perpetrators, often unknowingly. As consumers, we participate in the inhumane treatment of animals simply by purchasing certain foods and products derived from animals raised and slaughtered inhumanely. This agricide extends to the natural world as well, since the factory systems of livestock, poultry, fish, and wild animal production all lead to deadly environmental pollution.

How many of us have thought about the sources of our food? What does it take to put the juicy steak, fresh eggs, or tender slice of veal on our plates? What makes it possible to buy a fast food hamburger for 99 cents? Do we know the source of our inexpensive leather shoes, cosmetics, wool coats or fur-lined jackets?

Each one of us would be pained to know the truth about the production methods of our food and consumer goods. Behind this cornucopia of plentiful and inexpensive food and goods is a high price tag paid by the animal kingdom, the environment, and by developing countries whose human and natural resources are being plundered in order to meet Western societies' growing appetites. To live in denial of the

11

harmful consequences of many of our consumer choices, habits, and expectations is to deny our sensibilities for humane treatment of life, and ultimately, to deny our own well-being and survival as a species.

Kitchen Anarchists

Consumers can become "kitchen anarchists," simply by supporting local, humane organic farmers and market co-ops. This can begin by asking your local supermarkets and restaurants to offer organic foods, humanely raised meat, and vegetarian dishes as options. And if they do not carry these items, avoid these venues and take your consumer dollars elsewhere. Anarchy, when it comes to food and agriculture, begins with enlightened consumer choices. The Constitution secures what comes out of our mouths—freedom of speech—but it will be up to consumers to secure what goes into our mouths.

Bioethics is a new word for an old concept. It is the extension of ethical issues and concerns from the immediate human community into the broader biological dimension of our relations with, and duties toward, the biotic community—animals, plants, and the whole of nature. Bioethical principles in food production and consumption are the keys to a more sensible and compassionate future.

The bioethical basis for helping ensure food quality, safety, and security demands ethical consistency in the values and the decision making at all levels of food production. Food is sacred. Yet, some may ask, Why care? My response is that caring adds meaning to life, and most importantly, secures a future for life. Ethical behavior is one way I can show gratitude for the many blessings in my life and express my spirit of a reverential respect for all life.

There are still some farmers, ranchers, academics, policy makers, and consumer advocates who are willingly and eagerly working for the necessary counter-revolution in industrialized agriculture. They are helping to bring back food production that respects and restores the land. Eco-agriculture produces food that is safe and nutritious and at a fair price. With the support of consumers who demand and buy food from and for a healthy world, this revolution in agriculture can happen.

The Consumer's Right to Know

The pivotal issue of the industrialization of agriculture, referred to as agribusiness, is the consumer's right to determine who produces food and how. A handful of multinational corporations are gaining a monopolistic control over the entire food production system, from seed stock and breed stock to market shelf space. As long as food is cheap and plentiful, why should this concern urban consumers? There are many reasons, ranging from animal welfare and environmental concerns to consumer health and economic fallout. This book spells out those reasons.

Numbers are difficult to visualize, and can often be upsetting. Yet, in the United States alone, 7,000 calves, 130,000 cattle, 360,000 pigs, and 24 million chickens are killed every day in order to support a meat-based diet. If you can, imagine that the average American consumes approximately 2,400 animals in a lifetime. In order to satisfy this meat consumption, agribusiness has developed an immense slaughtering machine that causes great suffering to animals, creates long-term environmental disasters, endangers healthy food production, and ultimately, threatens the economic independence of developing countries who support this growing American appetite.

Our food production system, from farm to table, has become a big time, highly industrialized business—agribusiness. At a great cost to future generations, industrialization of food has resulted in the production of more food, in particular meat, than is actually needed in the developed world. Corporations eye third world countries as opportunities for furthering industrialization, claiming technology and mass consumerism in the world market will help poor and struggling nations. Many developing countries have expanded their animal production for export, while their people go hungry. For example, in Guatemala, over half the children under five are starving, yet their country exports tens of millions of pounds of meat each year to the United States.[1]

Farmers, consumers, and environmentalists have many different values and concerns; however, we all share one thing: We eat. Food is the common ground. The healthfulness of that food ultimately depends on informed consumers and where they choose to spend their money in the marketplace. In turn, this will influence agricultural decisions made by farmers and by the food industry. Yet, as it stands today, decisions in the food industry are mostly based on high levels of production, speedy turn around time, and maximum profit.

The humane treatment of animals or serious consideration of environmental effects of certain food production practices are given low priority in the decision-making process by agribusiness. Because of the decisions made by agribusiness, all of us are faced with widespread pesticide use and other agrichemicals sprayed on crops. As for animals, livestock production is based on inhumane factory conditions, bolstered by antibiotics, growth hormones, and chemical-based feed additives pumped into them daily. At this point in the earth's history, nearly all land, water, and air is contaminated with these substances. Few living beings are left unscathed. These harmful substances can be found in human mothers' milk and in fetal tissue, as well as in the reproductive and immunological systems of numerous other species, worldwide.

As a veterinary student in England some forty years ago, I worked on traditional farms. The animals included free-range sheep, dairy cows, poultry, pigs, and beef cattle. There were occasional instances of animal neglect by farmers, but these were made more from ignorance than indifference. The animals were free to be themselves, and most of the farmers had great affection for both their animals and the land.

In 1978 I walked into a "factory farm" for the first time. It was a small battery-hen egg factory. Soon after that I visited a small hog-confinement building. I was in a state of suspended disbelief, bordering on shock. In the nearly twenty years since then, I have visited much larger factories, dairy and beef cattle feedlots, as well as auction yards and slaughterhouses. I am still horrified by the inhumane treatment of animals and still shocked by the unhealthy conditions for humans and the environment. I also have seen the ravaged ranges of the Southwest due to livestock overgrazing, as well as those of India and East Africa. In these places, the vitality of the land has become as lifeless as the eye of a tethered sow or a high-tech factory dairy cow.

I cannot believe that those who were once farmers—though some have resisted and thousands more have gone out of business—could ever consider adopting such cruel "intensive" methods of animal production. In order to do so, these high-tech "farmers" must sever their empathy for the animals and treat them as "production units," biological machines. Now, agribusiness calls its farmers "producers" and "contract growers." Sad, but accurate, titles. Most of today's food growers are not farmers, but rather people who have been co-opted into the industrialization of agriculture.

There are still caring farmers and ranchers, yet they, too, are becoming endangered. In today's corporate agribusiness system the caring farmer is becoming an endangered species replaced by contract growers or corporate serfs. Family farmers and ranchers who wish to practice humane sustainable farming are unable to compete with the behemoth of industrial agriculture. During the past decade, we have witnessed the demise of hundreds of thousands of family farms and ranches. The seeds of wisdom, passed on from generation to generation by family farmers and ranchers, are being lost forever as these people leave the land. Inevitably much of their land will become part of large factory farms for industrialized food and livestock feed production.

Food production in the United States, and in many other countries, has become a system that has no respect for life—only for profits. If people kept their pets under conditions similar to those for factory farm animals, they would be in violation of state animal protection laws. But because these living beings are only "farm animals" destined to be consumed, the quality of their existence is of little concern to most. This agricide continues in large part due to the fact that most consumers are unaware, uninformed, and disconnected from the land and the sources of their food.

Productivity and efficiency are the higher goals of the industrial agricultural economists, agronomists, and animal production scientists who dismiss the cruel incarceration of animals, abuse of the land, and widespread pollution of the food chain as the price of progress. In the end, agribusiness places the blame on consumers, claiming that their demand for cheap food forces agribusiness to adopt such practices. Industrialization of food has made agriculture nonsustainable by breaking the connections between the health and well-being of farmers, consumers, farm animals, and the land itself. Conventional industrial agriculture, as well as aquaculture (factory farming of fish), are contributing substantially to the earth becoming a bioindustrialized wasteland that will impoverish future generations in both body and spirit.

Whom Can You Trust?

Unfortunately and unnecessarily, our food is neither safe nor cheap. My concern is that we will soon find it impossible to sustain a plentiful supply of wholesome food. With the advent of genetic-engineering biotechnology, agribusiness corporations are creating food that comes from farmerless fields and fieldless foods—far removed from nature's cycles and seasons for growing food. These same corporations are already producing "designer foods," composed of synthetic ingredients. They have engineered disease and herbicide-resistant seeds that already contain their own pesticides.

The consequences of this unfeeling approach to the earth are already being felt. We have witnessed epidemics of bacterial food poisoning so severe in the United States that the government now plans to irradiate chicken, pork, and other foods. In addition, there is an ever-increasing loss of topsoil and vital soil nutrients, compounded by escalating environmental contamination. This is especially apparent in ground water and drinking water contaminated by excessive use of chemicals in farming, along with excessive animal waste with its high levels of nitrogen, phosphates, and bacteria.

The proliferation of huge factory farms and feedlots spreads the blight. Corporations have gained a monopolistic control over agriculture from field to table. Corporate agribusiness reduces competition, controls prices, and prevents the adoption of more equitable, humane, and environmentally sound agricultural systems. Agribusiness veils the hidden costs of big business farming behind rhetoric that proclaims America has the safest, cheapest, and most plentiful supply of food in the world.

As a consumer, it is difficult to know whom to trust. In recent years, I have asked many questions as I watched the phenomenon of big business take over the food industry. In turn, I ask you these same questions.

♦ Would you trust any government that refuses to enforce labeling of genetically engineered food and denies consumers the right to know if any food they buy is not natural? The United States Federal Drug Administration has refused to enforce such labeling.

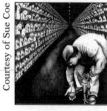

Courtesy of Sue Coe

♦ Is it possible to believe factory farming experts who say four or five laying hens in a cage 18 inches by 24 inches do not really suffer? Or that veal calves in narrow crates and mother sows in narrow stalls do not really need to turn around or walk or feel the sun on their backs? Some 90 percent of the meat eaten by Americans today comes from animals grown in a factory farm or feedlot environment, where these conditions are commonplace.

Why Eat with Conscience?

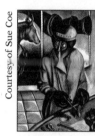

Courtesy of Sue Coe

♦ Would you support a livestock industry that sees nothing wrong with feeding farm animals the remains of livestock classified at the slaughterhouse as already dead, dying, diseased, or debilitated? In the United States, forty billion pounds of this "offal" are fed back to farm animals annually, which will eventually be consumed by humans who eat their meat, eggs, and milk.

♦ Can you trust the technophiles of industrial agriculture who say that the efficiency of factory farms is the answer to feeding the poor and hungry of the world? This is the same industry that has put out of business tens of thousands of self-sustaining small farmers and their families, not only in this country, but worldwide—all in the name of progress and profitability.

♦ Can you believe a livestock industry and their technical experts who see nothing wrong with feeding antibiotics every day to farm animals, knowing the grave risks of antibiotic-resistant bacteria to the consumer public? Agribusiness claims antibiotics are necessary in order to reduce consumers' and farmers' costs because sick animals are less productive and grow slowly. However, antibiotic-resistant infections are increasing at an alarming rate among humans, especially among infants, the elderly, and those with compromised immune systems.

During the past two decades of working in animal welfare and reform, I have heard the lies, denial, ridicule, and concerted opposition of the agribusiness establishment. The powers that be want to maintain the status quo of intensive, industrialized animal agriculture to further the economic interests of a powerful few. The many hidden costs are neither revealed to the public nor to company shareholders. These hidden costs include extensive government subsidies in feedstuffs, and low-interest loans from the federal government and from banks to factory farmers who want more confinement buildings for livestock or farm equipment. Consumers and taxpayers also pay for environmental damages due to surface and ground water pollution. Corporate agribusinesses also do not divulge the high costs of animal health problems and death because of inhumane treatment to livestock.

In turn, the agribusiness establishment also denies the role of ani-mal-based agriculture in contributing to increased consumer health problems. Agribusiness would like the consumer to believe that plenty of meat and milk in the daily diet is beneficial when in fact numerous scientific studies directly relate cancer and other diseases to a high consumption of meat and animal fat.

Unfortunately, the list of doubts will only continue to grow as we enter the next millennium. In the past fifteen years, there has been an increasing incidence of livestock and poultry health problems as more intensive "factory" farming systems become the norm. England has already faced mad cow disease and the resulting illness and death to both humans and animals. The fallout from mad cow disease continues to take its toll in England. Richard Rhoades predicts in his book, *Deadly Feasts*, that the United States is just a few years behind England in grappling with its own epidemic.

Making a Difference

As a child growing up in early post-World War II England, I remember the wonder and delight of skylarks singing over golden wheat fields. The silver morning mists that moved silently in the breeze across old cow pastures enthralled me. In these meadows, my dog and I found all kinds of fascinating creatures—voles, rabbits, lizards. Scarlet pimpernels and wild forget-me-nots bloomed along the perime-ters of the wheat fields, and daisies, buttercups, brambles and wild roses joined one another in the meadows. There were ponds, too, on this half-wild farmland, teeming with life, and from which the cows drank. Our milk, eggs, butter, vegetables, fruit, and meat came from this farm. The farmer, Mr. Holgate, often delivered the produce himself to our small suburban community in the north of England.

The farm is gone. My memories now lie buried under a middle-class housing development. It is nostalgia, I know, but I long for the beauty, biodiversity, and ecological integrity of Mr. Holgate's farm. Can farms such as these, alive with nature's fullness and spontaneity, be restored in a world besieged by human need and greed?

Fortunately, there are areas of our earth that still contain ecological diversity. There are communities that can support the Mr. Holgates of today. There are still signs of nature in places like Iowa and Vermont, and in many other farming regions of the world. Precious fragments of wildness and wilderness still remain. We can preserve these as well as restore areas that have been blighted. Prairies, savannas, wetlands, highlands, and woodlands on every continent can be revived, which will help prevent floods and soil erosion. And indirectly, restoring natural areas will provide natural pest controls for nearby crops because of the diversity in wildlife.

Individual consumers need to recognize that each one of us can make a difference in restoring the natural environment and supporting humane farming practices. When we re-establish our connection to the land and know the value of this connection, then we will be more willing to act on the environment's behalf as well as on our own. As more information becomes available that enables consumers to better understand the real costs of industrial agriculture, we can make informed choices—literally voting with our forks. Consumers can provide the necessary impetus for a profound change in agricultural production practices.

When individuals make a point to buy food that is humanely grown—whether it is animals or crops—this action supports organic and sustainable farmers and ranchers who are also trying to make a difference. Consumers can also support food retailers and public policy makers who are committed to a vision of a humane and sustainable agriculture.

In the United States, some 36.5 million acres of agricultural land have been set aside in the Conservation Reserve Program (CRP). This is part of a nationwide effort to restore nature and create a healthier rural environment. Simple steps such as planting grasses and trees along waterways on fields and along river edges will help stop soil erosion, chemical runoff, and provide wildlife cover. However, these simple steps, by themselves, are not enough. Farmers must change harmful agricultural practices and individuals must learn to consume healthier foods before real change can come about.

We might be too selfish a species to protect nature for nature's sake, but we can do so at least for our own sakes and for the future of our daughters and sons. Our own health and economic well-being are dependent upon thriving ecosystems. Healthy forests, wetlands, grasslands, and waterways mean healthy soils, crops, and air.

If we denature the environment, we undermine the economic value of the land. Basing public policy and agricultural practices on ecological economics is in everyone's best interest. It entails acknowledging the long-term astronomical economic savings of preventing water and air pollution, and soil degradation and loss. In turn, there are inestimable health benefits and health care savings by consuming foods grown in healthy soils, pure water, and a clean environment.

If reverence is sentiment, then we must be sentimental. If nostalgia is connectedness, then we must be nostalgic. Scientific agriculturists, like most other technocrats, reject sentimentality and nostalgia, just as they reject any feeling that softens them into considering more humane treatment of factory farm animals. But the wasteland need not spread. We can live in nature's image—the *imago dei*—that I sensed as a child.

Chapter Two

Factory Farming

A Holocaust in the Animal Kingdom

*From the beginnings of domestication of animals, interest
in their freedom from suffering has been subordinated to
economic considerations...But with the advent of factory
farming, the evil has been terribly accentuated.*

John B. Cobb, theologian

Traditionally, farm animals had the freedom to graze in open fields,
root in the soil, and wander about pecking in the farmyard. They
cared for their young in natural, comfortable farm surroundings, and
in turn, the farmers respectfully—and oftentimes lovingly—cared for
the animals. But all of that has changed.

For more than twenty years, I have been addressing a variety of
animal welfare issues that modern intensive methods of animal production—factory farms—have created in the quest for cost-saving "effi-
ciencies," higher production, and ever more profits.

Who owns these animal factory farms? Contract farmers usually
bear the mortgage and title to the operation. Yet, the ultimate con-
troller is the corporation that contracts to take all the products from
the farms for processing, and marketing to the public. Farmers pay the
bank, but their profit margins shrink as interest rates on loans
increase. Farmers keep going like a mouse on a treadmill while the corporations reap greater profits from high productivity and benefit more
than farmers from generous government subsidies. (See Chapter Three
on government subsidies.)

Who Benefits from Factory Farms?

There is a widespread lack of understanding of how consumer
habits and farming practices affect the animal kingdom. This is partly

because the majority of people live in urban environments and generally are not involved in the raising, catching, harvesting, killing, processing, or even preparation of their own food. It is essential that consumers become informed so that they can provide the necessary impetus for a profound change in agricultural production practices. Only when consumers begin to make conscious choices will the marketplace change.

Factory farming systems have increased in size over the past decade in spite of concerted national and international efforts to put an end to them. Although farms and ranches have reduced in number,

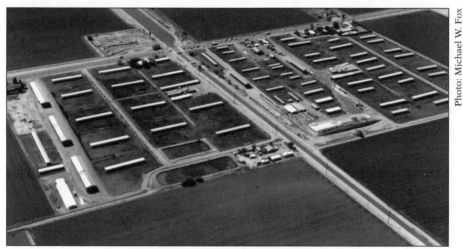

Photo: Michael W. Fox

Dairy factory farm in Arizona.

they have increased in size. For instance, beef cattle feedlots now typically have fifty thousand to one hundred thousand animals incarcerated in poorly drained dirt yards with neither shade nor shelter. In many cases, dairy cow herds of three thousand to five thousand head suffer the same conditions. These big business farms are now so commonplace that only about 10 percent to 15 percent of our meat, dairy, and poultry products come from smaller "family" farm operations. If this trend continues, some fifty thousand or so mega-farm complexes will be the main source of consumables for U.S. consumers and for export markets. This situation is a far cry from the four million family farms and ranches that fed the nation only twenty years ago.

The costs of intensive animal production far exceed the benefits. Industry spokespersons claim that consumers benefit from a cheap and

plentiful supply of animal products. However, the true primary beneficiaries are agribusiness corporations, especially food processors, animal-feed wholesalers, and drug and agrichemical manufacturers. What
benefits accrue to the consumers from industrial agriculture are
insignificant compared to the plethora of hidden costs.

Estimated Inputs Used to Produce Each Pound of Meat, Eggs, and Milk in the United States*

	Grain (pounds)	Energy (gals. gasoline)	Water (gallons)
Pork	6.9	0.44	430
Beef	4.8	0.25	390
Chicken	2.8	0.19	375
Eggs	2.6	0.14	n/a
Milk	0.1	0.02	n/a

Meat measured in boneless, trimmed weight. Includes soybean meal.
The energy equivalent of a gallon of gasoline is used only for convenience.
Most of the energy consumed is natural gas used in fertilizer production.

Sources: Grain from Cattle-Fax. Englewood, Colorado except for eggs and
milk based on data from U.S. Department of Agriculture; energy from David
Pimentel, Cornell University, Ithaca, N.Y.; Water from Jim Oltjen, University
of California, Davis.

*Alan Durning. "Fat of the Land." *World Watch 4.* May-June 1991.

About one-half of all the energy used in American agriculture goes
into livestock production for meat. The market price of meat and eggs
does not fairly reflect the costs of the grain, energy, and water used to
produce them. (See table above on estimated inputs.)

Beef, pork, and poultry from intensive production systems clearly
entail an incredible expenditure of energy. Livestock farming based on
forages such as alfalfa and highly nutritious grasses, is infinitely more
efficient, ecological, and profitable than conventional intensive confinement production. An energy tax on chemical fertilizers would help
reduce the wastefulness of such systems by encouraging farmers to
feed less grain and soybeans and more forages to these animals. But
feeding more forages produces more methane gas. (See section, Cattle
Methane and Global Warming, later in this chapter.) The answer must

come from consumers who simply choose to eat less or no meat, and buy natural, organic foods.

Hidden Costs of Factory Farms

As you can well imagine, supermarket prices do not reflect a fair and full-cost accounting of the food we buy. The real costs are hidden from the consumer. In almost every instance consumers pay the expense of doing business in industrial agriculture. The real costs of factory farming range from government price supports and subsidies at taxpayers' expense, to the demise of small family farms and rural communities, waste of natural resources, environmental pollution, animal stress, disease, and suffering.[1] The federal government uses taxpayer dollars to subsidize pesticides, irrigation, animal-feed costs, waste-management costs, and disease control. These costs are tax-deductible business expenses, enabling agribusiness corporations to save even more money. Examples of direct business costs that are tax deductible include crop losses, animal diseases that lower productivity, and high animal mortalities. The CEO of one major agribusiness conglomerate confided to me, "Farm animal welfare is not a moral or ethical issue. It's an economic one."

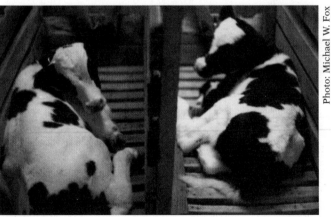

Photo: Michael W. Fox

Veal calves in crates can neither walk nor turn around.

I call this line of reasoning *economism*—doing business without regard for moral or ethical concerns such as animal suffering, environmental impact, or consumer health. With economism, farmers do not believe they can afford, in a competitive world, to consider concerns such as animals' well-being if competitors do not do so too. Consequently, we all become the victims and perpetrators of a competitive downward spiral.

Consumers pay higher health care costs because they eat foods treated with excessive pesticides and antibiotics, as well as experience the effects of over-consumption of a diet too high in animal fat and protein. Long-term costs to future generations, like topsoil loss and drinking water contamination, are also not accounted for, nor are the calories of fossil fuel and gallons of water required to bring each product from field to table.

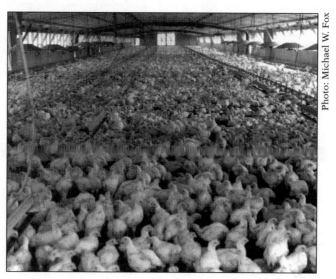

Photo: Michael W. Fox

A typically overcrowded broiler chicken unit.

Animals as Production Units

The cruelest fallout from the industrialization of agriculture is the treatment of farm animals, now coldly referred to as "production units." One particularly gruesome example of inhumane farming is that most gourmet, milk-fed veal comes from calves raised in almost complete isolation for sixteen weeks. They live in narrow crates where they can neither walk, turn around, nor comfortably lie down. They are fed a liquid diet laced with antibiotics and low in iron to keep their flesh pale. In a further effort to keep their flesh pale, the calves are kept in a state of borderline anemia by depriving them of hay and roughage, which they crave.

Another example of cruel factory farming is the extremely abusive practices used in commercial egg houses. More than 90 percent of the eggs we consume come from laying hens that live in a cage with a floor space only about twice the dimensions of a regular phone book. Four or five hens share this space. There is not enough room for the hens to lie down, fluff their feathers, or even stretch their wings. Because of the cramped

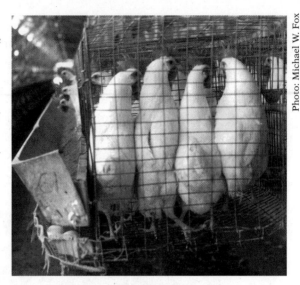

Laying hens in a factory farm.

cages, chickens become crazed, pecking one another severely, sometimes to death. Poultry producers solve this problem by "de-beaking" the chicks with hot knife machines—a procedure considered painful by anyone who believes animals can feel.[2]

In many commercial sheds, seventy thousand to one hundred thousand or more laying hens or broilers (raised for meat) crowd together under one roof. Diseases and infestations often sweep through the flocks at an alarming speed and require extraordinary applications of various drugs and toxic chemicals. A Maryland farmer, who now farms organically, told me that commercial egg factories hyperstimulate young hens with artificial light to get them to start laying eggs before they are fully grown. The industry uses the term "blowout" to describe what happens to some of these hens when they are forced to lay too early—the hens' vents (posteriors) burst, and they die. Broiler flocks have sometimes gone crazy, and in wave upon wave, bash themselves to death in mass hysteria inside the poultry shed. A Virginia farmer first told me of these things in 1976. He said that hearing seventy thousand birds becoming one mad wave of feathers, excrement, and death almost drove him crazy too. Furthermore, hens are starved for up to thirty hours before they are slaughtered. Poultry producers reason that any food given during this time would not be converted to flesh, and therefore a waste.[3]

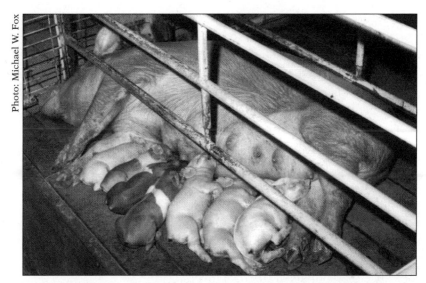

Photo: Michael W. Fox

A narrow birthing crate is supposed to prevent the sow from lying on her piglets, but she often does because she cannot turn around.

Pigs also fall prey to industrial agriculture practices of intensive confinement. Most pork, ham, and bacon come from corn-fed pigs whose mother sows live in gestation and farrowing (nursing) crates in which they can never walk or turn around as long as they live. Modern farm methods for pigs often include taking the piglets away from their mothers soon after birth. This results in a forced weaning, which allows the sow to end her lactating period so she can become pregnant again. And in order to reduce piglet death due to emotional loss, they may be given a mechanical teat as a substitute. The mother's emotional loss is a nonissue.

Hundreds of breeding sows and thousands of fattening piglets live in small, cramped pens in long, unheated, often poorly ventilated sheds. They never feel warm sunlight on their backs or natural dirt beneath their hooves. When all the natural instincts are removed, the pigs become bored, frustrated, and are driven to gnaw neurotically on one another's tails and hind ends. The pig producers' solution to this problem is to routinely amputate the pigs' tails.[4]

Journalist David Nevin of the *Smithsonian Magazine* (April 1980) interviewed me about farm animal welfare problems and animals' rights. During the interview, we met a Virginia hog farmer who was one of the first in his county to raise hogs in confinement, but quit factory farming after a horrendous accident. He lost a batch of pigs when the building in which they were confined exploded. Apparently, there was a gas buildup in the manure pits under the slatted floors of the pig barn. "It was a hell of a mess," the farmer recalled. "There were bits of pig everywhere. I never went back to total confinement after that."

Once farmers push animals' productivity too far, disease incidence increases. Effects of overfeeding high-energy "concentrates" to dairy cows and beef cattle contribute significantly to a variety of health problems. These include fatty liver disease, mastitis, crippling foot diseases, and overall weakening of the immune system, which result in higher incidence of infectious diseases. Hogs and poultry also suffer from a variety of other so-called "production-related diseases."

Investigators found a high incidence of gastric erosion in cattle fattened on rations containing corn—33 percent—compared to a 3 percent incidence in cattle fattened on rations containing no corn.[5] In fattening hogs, corn meal ground too fine to facilitate digestion is a major cause of esophageal (throat) ulcers.

Another serious problem for animals raised in confinement is the buildup of thick layers of fecal material on their hides, often weighing several pounds. This fecal mass especially accumulates around their thighs, tails, and genitals. Bacteria and acids in the manure actually eat away at the hide, with the skin wearing away to expose raw nerve endings. This is terribly painful for the animals. And this can be a major source of bacterial contamination of carcasses at slaughter.

Cows are ruminants, having evolved to make their way on grass and forage, not on high-energy grain fed to increase milk production. As a result of this forced diet, their digestive tracts rebel continuously giving them a perpetual case of diarrhea that coats their tails in multiple layers of manure. The response of many farmers is to simply cut off the tails, which is the cow's only natural protection against flies. These cruel and unnecessary cow mutilations occur on family farms that have as few as forty head of cattle, as well as on the mega-farms that have hundreds of milkers. I believe that cow-tail bobbing is a sign of a desperate farmer and an abusive society.

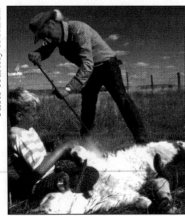

Photo courtesy of FARM.

Hot-iron branding of cattle is unnecessary.

Hot-iron branding of cattle causes considerable suffering, yet it is a common practice in the United States, although illegal in some countries such as the United Kingdom. Cattle states like Colorado and Texas still mandate hot-iron branding of cattle, even though humane alternatives like ear tags and microchip implants work just as well. The U.S. federal government mandated that Mexico brand millions of its cattle on the side of the face before allowing the animals to be imported. The United States Department of Agriculture (USDA) did not make any effort to change this barbaric practice until late in 1994.

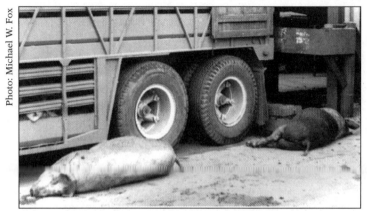

Photo: Michael W. Fox

Dead hogs due to the stress of transportation.

When animals are transported for slaughter, of every one hundred animals marketed, seven to nine have severe bruises, a clear indication of inhumane treatment.[6] Livestock are often transported for many hours. Under federal law they are supposed to be given rest, food, and water every twenty-eight hours while in transit. This is too long a time between water and feed intervals. However, this law only applies to transport by rail, whereas most animals are shipped by truck. The livestock industry loses $46 million annually from bruises on cattle and hogs. Federal inspectors condemn this bruised meat, enough to feed a large city, *but only if they see it*, during cursory visual inspection.

Annually, the United States pork industry loses $32 million from stress-prone hogs whose meat becomes unfit for marketing. Stress in pigs results in "pale-soft-exudative" meat or "PSE meat" as a result of transportation stress. Of the ninety million pigs slaughtered every year, some two hundred thousand pigs are condemned for human consumption due to disease, abscesses, and being dead on arrival at the packing plant. Thirty-seven percent of defective hogs are dead upon arrival due to poor handling and transport methods.[7]

The USDA documented the unintentional death of 4.37 million cattle and calves in 1991. The estimated economic losses were about $2.1 billion. The national average for calf mortality is about 3.5 million animals per year, worth some $850 million. This is a reflection of poor husbandry practices.[8] In January 1997 *Beef Today* magazine reported that in the United States annually, approximately 2.7 million calves die before reaching one month of age.

Few livestock specialists are outspoken on animal welfare issues, but one exception is Pennsylvania State Extension Swine Specialist Kenneth B. Kephart. In his *Pork Prose* column, he states:

> **If we totaled all the marketing losses nationwide, we'd find that over 250 hogs show up dead at packing plants every day. That's more than we could fit on one tractor-trailer load and amounts to about $27,000. Although most of these deaths are probably avoidable, the industry regards them as acceptable.**
>
> **Death losses during transport are too high—amounting to more than $8 million per year. But, it doesn't take a lot of imagination to figure out why we load as many hogs on a truck as we do. It's cheaper. Even with a zero death rate associated with more space on the truck, the hogs that we save would not be enough to pay for the increased transportation costs of hauling fewer hogs per load. So it becomes a moral issue. Is it right to overload trucks and save $.25 per head in the process, while the overcrowding contributes to the deaths of 80,000 hogs each year?[9]**

With factory farming there is no heart and no soul connection with the animals raised for food. Industrialized livestock and poultry producers think of and treat animals as though they are unfeeling machines. They have become mechanomorphized. Recently, at a state Pork Producers Congress I debated a "pig expert" on the question of farm animal rights and farm animal welfare. He is a well-known farm animal production scientist and state university professor. I asked him if he thought pigs have feelings. He paused and then after some thought, cautiously said, "I think that they might have but I'm not sure. We need to do more scientific research before we can really know."

I must emphasize that many veterinarians vehemently oppose factory farming, and the American Veterinary Holistic Medical Association and the Association of Veterinarians for Animal Rights are actively promoting humane reforms. Furthermore, most farmers who have adopted factory systems of intensive livestock and poultry production are not doing it because they are cruel and indifferent. They have simply become caught up in the same cruel economic treadmill that they think justifies factory farming.

No other Western society, past or present, raises and kills more animals just for their meat to the degree that we see in the United States. But as other nations have industrialized they too have adopted such intensive systems of animal production and nonrenewable resource-dependent farming practices. These have evolved to meet the public expectation and demand for a cheap and plentiful supply of meat. The livestock industry depends on costly nonrenewable natural resources and precious farmland to raise the feed for these animals to convert into meat.[10]

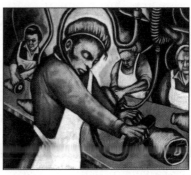

Courtesy of Sue Coe

To a hungry world, such conspicuous consumption is a poor, inefficient, and unethical model to emulate. This is the farmland that we could use more economically *to feed people directly* by raising highly nutritious crops such as cereals, legumes, and nuts for human consumption rather than using so much good land to fatten farm animals.

Supporters of intensive animal factory farming claim that the United States has the cheapest and most productive agriculture in the world. They insist that humane animal reforms will increase costs and put an unfair burden on the poor. Some people often think of critics of factory farming as being more concerned about animals than people and against progress. These are erroneous beliefs and conclusions. It is possible to care about both animals and people.

Disease and Drugs on Factory Farms

Producers need to increase revenue as production costs escalate. This is just sound business practice. Unfortunately, with agribusiness it has encouraged the adoption of large scale, intensive methods of livestock and poultry production. Producers now use drugs and chemicals to increase growth and food conversion efficiency. It is no surprise that 80 percent of all farm animals receive drug treatment. In a routine United States Department of Agriculture (USDA) survey in 1990, 15 percent of 1,946 meat samples contained new drugs they could not identify.

One estimate of the total death and disease losses in United States livestock is about $4.6 billion annually.[11] The United States Government Office of Technology Assessment more recently put this estimate up to $17 billion per year. Loss from pneumonia in hogs and cattle is about $800 million. In 1991 economic losses from respiratory diseases in cattle were $624 million, and $395 million from digestive problems. Pneumonia is a significant occupational health and safety hazard for people as well who work in poultry and hog-confinement operations. About 60 percent of employees in hog factories have at least one respiratory ailment.

Particularly disturbing are animal deaths attributed to calving or birthing difficulties. Poor nutrition, caused by inadequate forage or supplements, is the major reason cows do not rebreed, or rebreed late in the breeding season. In addition, farmers could prevent 60 percent of calf losses by giving timely and proper assistance to cows experiencing calving difficulties. Assistance also reduces rebreeding difficulties and promotes healthier mothers.

Milk production on factory farms causes a great deal of suffering to cows. Mastitis in dairy cows costs producers over $2 billion per year. And milk condemned because of antibiotic residues in factory cows treated for mastitis costs the dairy industry $50 million per year. Dairy cows grazing in green pastures once enjoyed a healthy productive life of twelve to fifteen years. Today, the modern factory farm pushes cows into high gear milk production that literally burns them out by two to three years of age. Thirty to 40 percent of the hamburgers eaten in the United States come from the slaughter of these burned-out, used-up dairy cows. Often the meat contains unapproved antibiotics and other drugs that producers use to extract the last gallon of milk out of the cows before they are slaughtered. The end result is milk laced with antibiotics and loaded with dead white blood cells (pus).

Lameness in dairy cows is another serious problem in factory farming. In part, crippling lameness is due to intentional overfeeding that causes rapid growth and bodies too heavy for the immature bones to support. Also, lack of sunlight in confined animals can aggravate lameness, especially in winter. Generalized metabolic bone disorders are common in factory cows. Revenue loss in dairy cattle due to lameness is more than $45 million annually in the United Kingdom. Annual losses from crippling lameness in confinement-raised hogs was more than $24 million for 1988 to 1989 in the United States.

Overcrowding on factory farms can also result in mange, a skin parasite that can cause considerable suffering. Mange spreads like wildfire when animals are in close contact and afflicts about 90 percent of swine herds in the United States.

Fifteen percent of live-born pigs die before weaning.[12] The pigs' mean age at death is six days. The most frequently reported instance of death in unweaned pigs (43 percent) was being crushed by the sow. This is not surprising given the minimal space allotted for the sow and piglets in birthing crates. Other reported instances of pig death, in order of reported frequency, include starvation, diarrhea, lameness or joint problems, deformities, respiratory illness, and nervous-system illnesses. More than 80 percent of the sampled farms maintained at least one confined farrowing (birthing) facility.

The broiler industry loses some $20 million from chickens dying from heart attacks every year because of the high stress of factory farm conditions and abnormally rapid growth rates. This is just one of a host of production-related diseases. Ascites, fluid accumulation under the skin, is another common affliction possibly linked with heart disease. Also, many broiler chickens develop painful arthritis and deformed limbs because they are bred and fed to grow abnormally fast. High humidity and ammonia levels burn the birds' lungs and eyes, and can lead to respiratory diseases and blindness in some instances. Other ailments include intestinal infections and skin burns called "breast blisters" that develop when the chickens lie down in their own excrement.

Blood-sucking northern fowl mites are a serious health and welfare issue that costs United States egg producers some $80 million a year.[13] Hens in battery cages are unable to easily preen and never can dust bathe. These are natural activities that help control these extremely irritating and debilitating parasites. Instead, chickens are often sprayed with pesticides and even fed the pesticides to control fly larvae developing in the piles of droppings under their cages.

The virtual immobility of laying hens in the crowded cages leads to osteoporosis. This causes their thin bones to fracture easily. When collected for slaughter, many hens suffer multiple fractures. In order to avoid broken bones in the meat, processing plant workers do not stun the birds by electrocution. The birds are fully conscious, terrified, and struggling on the shackle-conveyor when their throats are cut.

The Animal Health Institute reports that the total sales of United States animal health products were more than $2.2 billion in 1991, an increase of nearly 12 percent from 1990. Antibiotics for feed additives totaled $369.4 million in sales. Other feed additives such as drugs to control parasites totaled $226 million. Sales of veterinary products for use in livestock and poultry totaled over $150 million in 1989.

United States drug manufacturers produce more than thirty-one million pounds of antibiotics annually. Farmers feed nearly half of these antibiotics to farm animals. This results in *Salmonella* and other bacteria developing antibiotic resistance, a problem for both humans and farm animals.[14] The extensive use of antibiotics in the community, in hospitals, and as a food additive and disease prevention measure for factory animals has fueled what some predict will be a major health crisis in the next decade, namely, widespread bacterial resistance to antibiotics, our main defense against infections.[15]

Research at Iowa State University has discovered that antibiotic (tetracycline) resistant genes from pigs' manure can be passed on to soil bacteria and eventually find their way back to animals through soil-contaminated plants, and eventually to humans through the eating of the animals.[16]

The U.S. government justifies spending almost $4 million a year in public funds to help solve the costly animal health problems of the poultry and pig industries. This expense is especially troublesome since meat and poultry industries continue to justify, on false economic grounds of efficiency and productivity, the maintaining of such animals in overcrowded and unhealthy factory farms.

The 1995 estimate of medical costs and lost productivity from meat and poultry illnesses traced to seven foodborne human pathogens was $7.5 billion yearly, according to Robert Crutchfield, chief of USDA's Economic Research Service Food Safety Branch. Yet in the face of all these concerns and opposition from the Center for Disease Control and Prevention and consumer petitions, the USDA approved the routine use of a group of antibiotics called fluoroquinolones as a feed-additive by the poultry industry. Many human pathogens have not yet acquired resistance to fluoroquinolones; however, with continued overuse, it may only be a matter of time before this group of antibiotics becomes ineffective for human use.

As hog factories proliferate so does disease due to confined and crowded conditions. The practice of placing antibiotics in pig feed is now widespread because pork producers favor a fast-growing, "high-lean" variety of pig that is extremely susceptible to diseases. The only way for factory farm pork producers to stay in business is to continue to use antibiotics regularly.

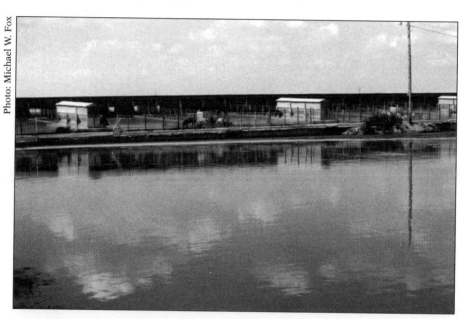

Photo: Michael W. Fox

Despite appearances, this livestock-waste holding "lagoon" on a factory farm is a major environmental problem.

Manure as Hazardous Waste

Enabling American farmers to feed far more animals than the regional land resources can sustain is not only detrimental to the developing countries producing the food for livestock, but also detrimental to the United States. It is unacceptable in part because of the tremendous amount of animal waste. The animal waste is not going back to the land from which the animal feed originated. Instead, animal manure has become a costly environmental management hazard and is a cardinal indicator of bad farming practices and defunct agricultural policy.

All agricultural practices receiving federal government support are presumably subject to critical and objective environmental impact assessments under the National Environmental Policy Act (NEPA). However, the U.S. government does not exercise its authority as empowered by this act. In many states, federal subsidies and price supports of various agricultural commodities and practices have had well-documented adverse environmental impacts. Enforcement of the NEPA would provide the incentive for farmers and ranchers to adopt less harmful practices, but there is neither the will nor interest in government and agribusiness to do so.

There are many bioregions in the United States that are subject to environmentally destructive and costly agricultural and livestock enterprises. The Chesapeake Bay ecosystem, for example, is being destroyed along with the livelihood and culture of the people who live and work there. The collective agrichemical runoff from fields and the animal wastes from highly concentrated livestock industries are the primary causes. Fecal bacteria from livestock contaminate the waters of Chesapeake Bay, and ultimately the seafood that can then cause food poisoning. Pesticides interfere with marine species' reproduction and immune systems, and may harm humans who eat the seafood. In addition, chemical fertilizers and manure disrupt the bay's ecology, causing proliferation of algae and potentially harmful microorganisms.

Opponents of factory farming were outraged by the provision in the 1996 Farm Bill to provide $200 million annually of taxpayers' money to help factory livestock operators handle animal manure more safely through containment lagoons. Several manure spills from poorly maintained hog factory and large dairy feedlot lagoons caused serious pollution problems in 1995, and this legislated remedy, on the surface, looked reasonable. However, critics see this provision as a subsidy to encourage and underwrite the proliferation of large confinement operations for livestock production.

Some of the worst manure spills were from hog factories in North Carolina, where North Carolina State University botanist Dr. Jo Ann Burkholder identified a lethal phytoplankton that proliferated in streams polluted by hog manure. This microscopic organism called *Pfiesteria piscidia* produces a powerful toxin that was responsible for massive fish kills in polluted waters.[17] This toxin can make people extremely ill, resulting in weight loss, abdominal cramps, festering sores, and memory loss. Phosphates in livestock manure stimulate this phytoplankton to bloom and is an example of the inherent dangers of animal (and human) waste in aquatic ecosystems.

Farmers have taken farm animals off the land, thereby breaking the nutrient manure cycle. Now farmers have to pay for more chemical fertilizers to replace the livestock manure. Consider the waste of shipping corn from Iowa to feedlots in Texas. The manure from the feedlot does not go back to enrich the depleted soils of Iowa. Instead, specialized, intensive livestock and poultry producers have a tremendous amount of unusable animal manure. If it is not managed correctly, it becomes a hazardous waste.

In areas where manure is put back into the soil, heavy metals, feed-additive chemicals, and pesticide residues, along with fecal bacteria, parasites, and residues of medications in the animals' feed, contaminate the land. These wastes from factory animal farms seep into the soil and groundwater and poison our lakes, rivers and coastal waters, and consequently the water we drink. Some 40 percent of the nitrogen and 35 percent of the phosphates contaminating the nation's rivers, lakes, and streams come from livestock wastes and feed fertilizers. For humans, nitrates in the drinking water can cause cancer. No one has yet determined the cost to clean animal wastes and agricultural chemical contaminants from our water supplies. However, the EPA does estimate that it will cost $2 billion to simply survey contaminated wells.

In many regions, excessive animal waste from factory farms is too much for the land to sustain. This is especially true where there are large concentrations of intensively raised livestock and poultry without a corresponding large area of farmland on which to spread the manure. In the United States, livestock and poultry excrete about 158 million tons of manure (dry weight basis) per year.[18] If we put this much manure in boxcars, the train would stretch around the world four and one-half times.

Much of this contaminated animal waste returns to the land to fertilize crops to feed these animals, which we then eat ourselves. Some farmers even feed the rendered remains of farm animals to their cattle, along with dried poultry manure. It is deplorable that livestock and poultry manure, once a vital nutrient resource in ecological farming, has become a hazardous waste in the factory farming system.

Eating with Conscience

In Europe, scientists are finding that manure gases contribute to acid rain, which is killing their forests. In U.S. poultry and hog confinement operations, dust and slurry vapors are an occupational safety hazard. They do not do much for the chickens' and pigs' health and well-being either, or for the well-being of downwind neighbors, whose property values plummet because of the stench. The smell alone often forces local residents to sell their homes because they lack the resources and government support to sue and stop these factory farms.

I grew up in the north of England where we had a saying, "Where there's muck, there's money." Now animal muck has become an environmental and public health hazard that contains enough excess nitrates to kill fish, pollute the environment, and pose serious human health problems. We also have to reckon with phosphates, various feed additives, and drugs in the animal manure, some of which may actually accumulate in crops from soils soaked year after year with slurry or contaminated manure. Fecal bacteria and other fecal organisms can survive in the soil for some time, get into surface waters, and ultimately into our drinking water. Witness the April 1993 Lake Michigan mess, when *Cryptosporidia* from livestock waste mismanagement caused more than a thousand people to get sick and everyone in Milwaukee had to boil their water for several days.

In some cases, instead of putting the manure back on the land, it is fed back to the animals. To the agricultural economist and animal production scientist, that might seem an efficient and innovative improvement on nature. However, health and environmental risks far outweigh any cost savings. A recent outbreak of botulism in Australian feedlot cattle that were fed poultry manure is evidence of the risks of mishandling animal waste. Chemical residues and drugs in poultry manure can make cattle sick. Sheep on pastures sprayed with pig slurry can develop copper poisoning. It is no surprise that the United Kingdom's Royal Agricultural Society concludes that animal manure from conventional factory farms that use drugs is too hazardous for use as a fertilizer, and that chemical fertilizers are safer.

Integrating livestock production systems with organic crop and forage production systems will lessen the likelihood of problem diseases. A major tenet of sustainable agriculture is that well-managed manure is a valuable resource, not a hazardous waste.

Trace Minerals and Impoverished Soils

Concerns about trace minerals may seem of little importance to consumers or farmers, but they point to a much larger and very serious problem: trace-nutrient deficiency diseases, about which we know very little. What we do know is that vital nutrients like selenium and zinc are essential for the immune system's ability to fight infections and for neutralizing harmful free radicals in cells that can cause cancer and other diseases. Our resistance to disease may be considerably impaired by the use of chemical fertilizers—simple phosphates, potash, and nitrogen—along with other farming practices like monocropping where farmers grow the same single crops on the same land year after year. These farming practices can result in the break of the molecular connections of the ecological food chain. The proper nutrients, especially trace minerals, needed to maintain the health of crops and all who eat these troubled harvests are not being returned to the soil. Instead of restoring the soil and testing it repeatedly, more business is made for the chemical and pharmaceutical industries as we must now add essential trace minerals to animals' feed and consumers are advised to take trace minerals as well.

Livestock producers use selenium, arsenic, copper, and zinc extensively as feed additives. These chemicals should not be considered relatively safe nutrients, like an amino acid or complex carbohydrate. They can be toxic to animals when improperly mixed, and toxic to other animals when they become concentrated in manure and fertilized forage.[19]

Chemicals such as selenium build up in the soil[20] as well as in surface and groundwater, in aquatic life, and subsequently in birds and land animals.[21] These chemicals even appear in certain plants[22] that farm animals consume, and in crops that humans consume[23] from fields fertilized with animal manure that contains these trace minerals.[24] Just as government regulates veterinary pharmaceuticals and nonveterinary drugs such as antibiotics and other feed additives, it must also strictly regulate trace-mineral feed additives such as selenium.

When the background level of a trace mineral is already high, the possibility of farm animals being overdosed and poisoned when feed manufacturers and growers add a trace nutrient to animals' feed is very real.[25] Sickness, impaired immunity, lower fertility, impaired growth rate, and decreased milk or egg production are some of the consequences. The toxicity of selenium and other chemical feed additives may be increased further when used with other additives or medications. This can promote widespread disaster. However, the feed additive industry claims to be "self-regulated" and the government maintains that regulating it is expensive and unfeasible.

It is incumbent upon the FDA and responsible farmers to treat selenium and other trace-element feed additives with the same degree of concern as antibiotics and growth hormones. We urgently need rigorous quantification of the evenness of selenium distribution in animal-feed formulation and processing. The U.S. government has eliminated the requirement for premix manufacturers to analyze effectively each production batch that contains selenium. There are no valid reasons for this. Likewise, there are no valid grounds for assuming that the same level of selenium in the premix is safe for food animals no matter where they live. Local FDA agents should quantify the presence of selenium in the animals' environment, including soil, water, feed, and forage. Then the manufacturer can make appropriate adjustments for the amount of selenium needed.

In the meantime, buying certified organic foods is the only safe bet because farmers who farm organically first ensure the restoration of the soil. A variety of organic crops have been found to contain far more essential trace minerals and vitamins than crops from conventional chemical farms, according to analyses done by biochemist Sharon B. Hornick of the Nature Farming Research and Development Foundation in Washington State.[26]

Animal and Human Hazards in the Slaughterhouse

For years I have witnessed factory farms, which look like a living hell for animals, with miserable working conditions for employees as well. Agribusiness companies that contract with "growers" to raise factory hogs or poultry or feedlot lamb and beef, rabbits and now ostriches and deer, often bring in cheap labor to work in their new slaughterhouses, now called "packing plants" (a sanitized term used by ConAgra, Cargill, British Petroleum, and other multinational corporate oligopolists). These corporations often get state and county tax breaks, promising the communities they invade plenty of new jobs, a new school, or perhaps a hospital annex. They then bring in cheap labor from Central America or Southeast Asia or employ locals at minimum wage with no health benefits or insurance programs. In turn, these employees are treated with the same lack of concern or compassion as the farm animals.

Major human welfare issues in the livestock and poultry industries are slaughterhouse and packing plant worker health, safety, and injury compensation. An era of neo-slavery exists in the major poultry and pork-producing states, such as North Carolina, Oklahoma, and Iowa. Investigations of the meat inspection system and of the handling and slaughter, as well as the transportation of livestock and poultry to the processing plants, underscore the urgent need for immediate state and federal correction.[29]

Current agricultural and economic policies have severely undermined the health of farm families as well as that of livestock and the environment. Kelley J. Donham, veterinarian and occupational health expert, points out—in vivid detail—congressional indifference to these problems. For example, he documents how hazardous it is to work in the foul air of hog factories where the poor pigs have no relief until slaughter. Workers develop serious chronic respiratory problems from poisonous gases and fecal "dust" particles.[30]

Standard conditions in even the best equipped slaughter and meat packing plants are neither safe nor hygienic. Across the nation, serious outbreaks of food poisoning are occurring due to contamination of meat from fecal bacteria. This attests to the fact that there are serious lapses in the effectiveness of the meat industry safety network. This serious disrepair is due primarily to government attempts to reduce the meat industry's costs by allowing animals to be slaughtered at such a fast rate that meat inspectors have no time to properly check each carcass. Compliance with appropriate humane and hygienic standards for workers and animals alike are lax for similar reasons.

Neglect of psychological as well as physical harm to farm workers handling large numbers of animals in confinement factories is apparent. According to British researcher Professor M.F. Seabrook, stockpersons working in factory farming systems often display disturbing changes in behavior and attitudes. His observations show that:

♦ Humans learn to accept poor treatment of animals;
♦ Stockpersons learn to ignore auditory and visual signals of livestock distress;
♦ Because of signal overload, stockpersons give selective attention while ignoring certain abnormal behaviors of animals;

♦ Aggression levels in stockpersons can increase significantly;

♦ Suppression of caring feelings may occur. This interferes with the stockperson's ability to care for animals that will be killed and eaten.[28]

Recently, I learned of a youth in England who worked in a village slaughterhouse. A pig escaped and he chased it and beat it brutally in public. He was arrested and tried for cruelty toward the animal. His defense was that it was the only way he could cope with killing animals every day—to treat them "as though they had no feelings at all."

There is mounting scientific evidence that when stockpersons and slaughterhouse workers express a negative attitude toward livestock, as a consequence, the animals experience a chronic state of stress. This stress reduces the number of offspring that sows produce, the number

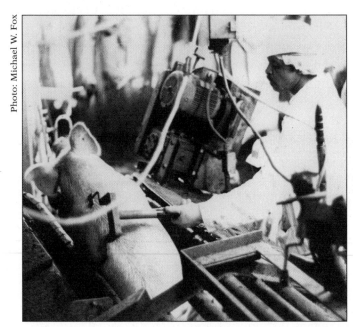

Photo: Michael W. Fox

Inhumane use of an electro-cution bar that should have been put across the pig's head. The pig is only paralyzed, not unconscious, as it should be prior to being slaugh-tered.

of eggs hens lay, and the amount of milk dairy cows give. Stress also affects growth rates and meat quality in broilers, piglets, and beef calves. In contrast, when farmers, farm workers, ranchers, and ranch hands treat animals gently, patiently and with understanding, the animals are healthier, more productive, and profitable.[27] However, mega-farms discount this fact in favor of the cost-savings of intensive livestock systems where one person is in charge of hundreds, even thousands of animals.

Mad Cow Disease and Animal Tankage

The bag of garden fertilizer proclaimed on a green stripe across its center: *Rich in Natural Organics*. I had bought the fertilizer to mix into the poor soil around the roots of some of my trees and perennial shrubs. Soon after I had cut the bag open and began to spread it, I got the dry heaves and had to stop. My acute attack of nausea took several minutes to subside.

I am no stranger to natural organic manure. I have shoveled tons of cow and pig manure on farms. Likewise, I have spread plenty of compost and organic bone and fish meal, and dry blood and seaweed on a variety of garden plants and kitchen crops. But never before have I become so sick so quickly by the smell of anything—except perhaps the smell of a rotting corpse. So I read the label of ingredients on the bag. Second to dried manure on the list of contents was *animal tankage*. I called the retailer. I correctly anticipated that the retailer had received no complaints from other users. This bag of garden fertilizer I had was so bad that I wondered if people have lost their common-sense olfactory wisdom. No one in their right mind would ever spread such noxious material around the house, where children and pets play, and where food is grown.

Animal tankage is the nonfat residue of unusable and condemned parts of livestock and poultry from slaughterhouses. The rendering plants slowly dry the tankage using low temperatures. Manufacturers add these byproducts (meat meal, or animal protein byproducts and bone meal) and tallow (animal fats that rise to the top of the rendering vats) to pet food as well as to livestock and poultry feed. *Beware: Read the ingredient label on your cat or dog food*. Chances are high that it contains rendered animal tankage, which may even include dead cats and dogs collected from animal shelters and veterinarians.

What better way for agribusiness to profitably dispose of so much factory farm hazardous waste—that amounts to forty-four billion pounds a year in the United States—than to turn it into animal feed and fertilizer? Seven million tons of animal tankage is fed to pets through the pet food industry in the United States annually. Animal tankage is also fed to food animals, including farmed shrimp and fish, and extensively used as fertilizer, potentially contaminating the fields and groundwater supplies.

Processed animal tankage is a potential source of bacterial and other contamination. This is partly due to the low-temperature processing procedure that does not always kill harmful organisms. Once added to livestock and poultry feed, animal tankage could contribute to widespread sickness and even death in the consumer populace. Animal tankage is potentially hazardous because it is a concentration of entrails, fecal material, bacteria, and various diseased and cancerous body parts. Through bioaccumulation, these inedible and condemned tissues and organs are contaminated with antibiotics, anabolic steroids, heavy metals, dioxins, long-acting pesticides and their hazardous metabolites. Perhaps by design, the U.S. government has virtually no health data available on the consequences of pesticide metabolites in the human body.

Farmers in the United Kingdom can no longer legally feed tankage to animals. Authorities in the United Kingdom destroyed nearly two hundred thousand cattle on sixteen hundred farms between 1992 and 1994 in an attempt to prevent the spread of a fatal degenerative brain disease called *bovine spongiform encephalopathy* (BSE) or "mad cow" disease. A virus-like organism called a "prion" is responsible for this disease. Prions are considered infectious proteins that do not evoke immune response, and can incubate within a living organism for years. To date, prions are considered the most lethal, self-perpetuating biological entities in the world. Prions are extremely heat-resistant and probably came from infected sheep brains in the animal tankage used in high-protein cattle feed.

The outbreak of BSE is one of the worst economic disasters in the livestock industry across Europe. Close to one quarter million afflicted and exposed animals were slaughtered because they had been fed potentially ineffective offal prior to 1988 when a ban was put on it in the United Kingdom for domestic use. Almost a million tons of beef, banned for consumption by humans, was put into cold storage in 1996. There was international outcry when other countries—notably France, a main buyer of British livestock feed, along with Thailand and Israel— learned that the United Kingdom had exported tens of thousands of tons of feed that may have been infected after the domestic ban had been imposed. There have been four hundred cases of BSE in

European cattle, so the disease has spread through exported feed from the United Kingdom. Since then, hundreds of cats in Europe and several zoo animals whose diets included animal tankage products have developed the brain disease. The feed ban in the United Kingdom did not stop this disease from being passed on to the calves of cows fed infected feed prior to the ban. This has raised further concerns that without slaughtering all dairy and beef cattle in the United Kingdom, the disease may never be contained and consumers will remain at risk.

There are doubts that cattle in the United States are free from BSE. Some of the thousands of so-called "downer" cows that go to slaughter every year may have this disease, manifested in a different form than in the United Kingdom. (Cows that are injured or become sick during transport to the stockyards or slaughterhouses are often too weak to stand and are called "downers." Dying, they are often pushed around by bulldozers into piles and left, sometimes for days, until dead.) The BSE tragedy in the United Kingdom should be a warning to the livestock industry worldwide. We cannot be feeding the remains of dead cows and other animals back to livestock.[31]

According to the USDA, more than ten million diseased, dead, dying, and debilitated cattle, calves, pigs, sheep, and lambs were rendered in 1995. The 282 rendering plants in the United States process forty billion pounds of offal, including two and one half billion pounds containing kitchen grease, the condemned parts of slaughtered livestock and poultry, liquids and scrapings from slaughterhouse floors, roadkill, and euthanized cats and dogs.

Of all rendered "animal proteins," approximately 10 percent is put into cattle feed, 36 percent fed to poultry, 15 percent to swine, and 36 percent about seven million tons—is put into pet food. I advise pet owners to read the labels on commercial pet food and avoid for obvious reasons those labels that say "meat byproducts" and "tallow." An excellent source for all pet owners and veterinarians is Ann N. Martin's book, *Food Pets Die For: Shocking Facts About Pet Food*. Martin documents what goes into most commercial pet food and the health problems that our pets can develop from such food.[32]

There is a strain of mad cow disease that affects humans, called Creutzfeld-Jakob disease. It can have a very long incubation period, often many years, before symptoms develop. Sixteen people have already contracted this disease in the United Kingdom. Infected animals and animal parts are potential health hazards. Products like hamburger, and garden and crop fertilizers, *rich in natural organics* (like the label on the bag of fertilizer) are also potential public health hazards. (For more information on Mad Cow Disease, see appendix.)

Cattle Methane and Global Warming

Some scientists are concerned that giving more forage to make cattle leaner will increase the amount of methane gas produced. Each cow emits from two hundred to four hundred quarts of methane gas daily. The world's cows contribute nearly fifty million metric tons of methane to the atmosphere every year. Methane is one of the gases associated with the trapping of infrared rays in the lower atmosphere that leads to global warming. Animal nutritionist Donald Johnson has suggested feeding antibiotics to cattle to kill some of the methane-producing bacteria in their rumen, or first stomach.[33] But even if this helps to reduce methane output by 30 percent and helps animals use their feed more efficiently, is administering more antibiotics the best solution?

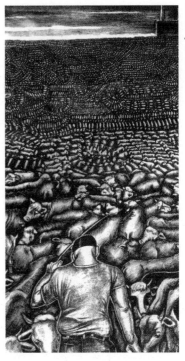

Courtesy of Sue Coe

Other animal scientists have proposed feeding livestock less forage and more grains.[34] But that's not the answer either, because the very practice of expanding grain production results in two greenhouse gases, methane and nitrous oxide, which are respectively absorbed *less* and released *more* from chemically fertilized and heavily cultivated land. Natural range land actually serves as a sink. It absorbs atmospheric carbon dioxide and the methane gas released by cattle and other ruminant animals. This helps offset the contribution of livestock to global warming. Chemically fertilizing and cultivating arable land to provide more grains for livestock will decrease methane uptake and increase nitrous oxide production, thereby contributing to the increasing atmospheric concentration of these gases. In turn, this will lead to increased global warming.[35]

The fact remains, however, that cattle do produce significant quantities of methane gas, as do the liquid manure lagoons adjacent to confinement livestock factories. One possible solution is to cover these lagoons to capture the bio-gas and generate energy. Some third world countries are adopting this practice. A few American dairy farmers are experimenting with methane-fired electric generators to provide electricity for their farms.

In 1992 the Center for Rural Affairs published a study on global warming and climate change entitled *Mares' Tails and Mackerel Scales*. According to the study, United States agriculture can reduce its contribution to greenhouse gas emissions by 28 percent through measures that will be good for farmers as well as for the environment. The report details strategies for reducing emissions from each major source. It concludes that the top priorities are to:

♦ Reduce nitrogen fertilizer use;

♦ Plant grass on highly erodible cultivated land;

♦ Reduce methane emissions from anaerobic lagoons where live stock waste decomposes without oxygen.

United States farms currently produce emissions of three major greenhouse gases that have the combined equivalent effect of about 643.6 million tons of carbon dioxide. Most startling is the finding that about one-fifth of all greenhouse gas emissions from major sources studied is from livestock waste that decomposes anaerobically in lagoons. Although only a small minority of farmers handle their animal waste this way, the percentage is growing as large-scale confinement facilities increase their share of the United States livestock market.

Simply, the most effective, long-term alternative to costly waste management systems is to eliminate having too many animals concentrated in one place. Factory farms are not the answer from an ecological perspective, as well as from humane and economic perspectives.

Environmental Costs of Factory Farms

The Federal Clean Water Act regulates pollution of surface waters in the United States, and considers concentrated animal feeding operations a source of pollution. Operators of livestock factory farms must obtain and install an expensive manure handling system. New or expanding facilities must also provide an Environmental Impact Statement. However, while most states have assumed responsibility for the Clean Water Act, there are serious concerns over lack of enforcement.

In 1993 several large factory farms and feedlots were operating or were under construction in states that, at that time, still did not require permits. For example, National Farms, which was the nation's largest hog farm but was recently sold to Premium Standard Farms, had built a sixteen-thousand-sow operation in the Texas panhandle. In the Oklahoma panhandle, Seaboard Corporation plans to construct a four million-head hog packing plant near Guymon. "Circle Four," a conglomerate of Smithfield Foods, Murphy Farms, Carroll Foods, and Prestige Farms, is planning a two-million pig factory farm in Utah.

While battles over new hog-raising facilities rage across the U.S., one of the nation's leading pork-producing firms, Carroll Foods, based in North Carolina, will build new hog factories in eastern Mexico's state of Veracruz, taking advantage of virtually nonexistent environmental regulations and cheap labor. The company says it will grow out six hundred thousand hogs per year at twelve locations. Carroll expects not only to supply markets in Mexico, but also to eventually export pork products to Japan.[36]

These factory farms are causing serious pollution and bacterial contamination of lakes, river basins, and drinking water. They have also caused several fish kills. Neighboring farmers and residents are filing lawsuits forcing the EPA to begin imposing costly livestock pollution controls since state authorities have refused to implement federal standards on their own.

The EPA estimates the costs involved in complying with the Federal Clean Water Act rules for these factory and feedlot operations as follows:

♦ $20,000 for a 200-head dairy operation;
♦ $40,000 for a 300-head beef feedlot or 750-head hog facility;
♦ $70,000 for a 1,000-head beef feedlot;
♦ $65,000 for a 2,500-head hog facility or 700-head dairy feedlot.

Most mega-farms have had a free ride in states that encourage the proliferation of such farms, in part because the costs of effective state and federal monitoring and enforcement are considerable. These are yet another hidden cost out of the taxpayers' pockets, all of which would be unnecessary if strict controls existed in the first place in every state to prevent mega-farm development.

One very good solution to these problems is to simply *reduce* the farm animal population to an environmentally and ecologically balanced number and distribution. A decrease in consumer demand for farm animal products is the key to this solution working. What we buy at the grocery store and put into our mouths has tremendous impact on the environment and animal kingdom it sustains. When consumers demand change with their food choices, their pocketbook, and their vote there will be an end to the production-consumption cycle of billions of animals worldwide. Animals who are forced to live in the disease-holes of intensive factory farms and feedlots that pollute the environment, put consumers at risk, and destroy rural communities.

Chapter Three

The Rotten Roots
of Agribusiness

*We do not inherit the land,
we borrow it from our children.*

anonymous

Some agricultural analysts conclude that there are too many farms in the United States. They say that small farms cannot compete with the big ones that have the advantage of so-called "economies of scale"—the bigger the better. Some people see traditional family farming as an outmoded institution whose passing is an inevitable consequence of progress.

It becomes easy in these circumstances to say the farm problem is simply due to poor management. This is exactly what happened during the bleak years of the Reagan administration, when, during the farm crisis of the 1980s, thousands of family farms went under. Reagan administration officials blamed the small farmers' crisis on poor management, thereby sweeping a national tragedy under the political rug. Hundreds of thousands of our nation's food providers had to leave the land and move into already crowded cities. A substantial segment of rural Americans faced disruption and financial ruin, and many of their lives ended in despair and suicide.

Family Farms Versus Corporate Agribusiness

Today, less than 2 percent of the people in the United States are farmers or ranchers. Yet they provide the food and fiber for the remaining 98 percent of our population. In contrast, in the days of Thomas Jefferson, some 80 percent of the population worked on the land. Without farmers and ranchers, we would be in dire straits.

With the advent of ever larger tractors, harvesters, and other farm equipment, the industrialization of agriculture intensified after World War II. It grew quickly thanks to chemical fertilizers and pesticides developed out of various governments' nerve gas experiments during the war. High-yield hybrid seeds also played a major role in the growing agribusiness industry. These advances set the stage for the demise of rural America and America's family farms.

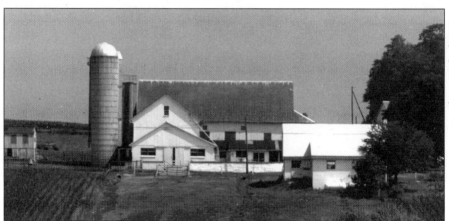

The family farm as Americans have known it in the United States is endangered.

Since around 1985, the plight of small farmers and ranchers has intensified. Between 1985 and 1990, more than 425,000 family farms have gone out of business. The agribusiness industry, especially via its magazines and journals, points a finger at animal rights' organizations as foes of the farmer and rancher. However, what is becoming apparent is that big business is the foe of the farmer and the rancher. In the 1990s, more and more farmers and ranchers are contacting animal rights' organizations as potential allies. Family farmers and ranchers are beginning to see themselves as victims of an indifferent agribusiness industry and government. The plight of factory farm animals ironically parallels the plight of the small farmer and rancher. They are all victims of the same highly competitive, economic treadmill that is indifferent to that which does not equate with bottom-line profit and market monopoly. As the animals have become mere commodities, so too have the family farmer and rancher become the expendable contract-labor of corporate feudalism.

The Rotten Roots of Agribusiness

A misinformed public perceives the small farmer benefiting from a plethora of subsidies. The truth is that subsidies to farmers only enable production to continue while the prices farmers receive at market do not cover most farmers' costs. The real beneficiaries of government subsidies are the agribusiness corporations that buy farm products at these subsidized low prices. For example, in 1997 $300 million was given to one U.S. grain company under the Agriculture Export Enhancement program to enhance its efforts for conducting business abroad. It is business as usual for the U.S. government to give millions of dollars to agribusiness corporations to underwrite their advertising costs for business overseas. In increasing numbers, small farmers and ranchers either go out of business or become contract growers for agribusiness corporations. Corporate managers dictate *how* and *what* farmers are to produce, resulting in what some observers—and some farmers themselves—term a new serfdom.

Very few people recognize or lament the loss of America's small family farms. Today the average age of U.S. farmers is fifty-five to fifty-six years. The economic structure is such that a younger, would-be farmer generation has little hope of ever farming except under corporate peonage as a contract grower. As a consequence, few choose to farm.[1]

When the family farm does not pass to the next generation, we lose traditional and indigenous knowledge, skills, cultural diversity, and democratic influence. Wisdom and love of the land become irrelevant when the family farm fails and becomes incorporated into the mega-factory farm. Regrettably, like natural biodiversity, the protection of cultural diversity, which includes the rural family life and sustainable social economics, is low on our national agenda.

Seventy percent of the nation's 2.2 million farms are noncommercial. They produce relatively small quantities of agricultural products and do not provide enough income to support a family, so off-farm jobs are the only way to make ends meet. Commercial farms with annual sales of more than $250,000 account for only about 6 percent of all farms. Yet this tiny number of American mega-farms account for a whopping 51 percent of all livestock sales and 55 percent of all agricultural sales.[2]

The transformation of agriculture into food industry oligopolies over which consumers will have neither choice nor control is now quickening. This loss of choice and control will probably be complete within the next decade if consumers do not support humane, sustainable agriculture. Few economic analysts and sociologists see the relationship between the demise of the family farm and rural life, and the increasingly dysfunctional state of the economy and urban life. Yet this connection is real.

Monopolistic Food Industry

In the United States, both the farming and the meat industry are controlled by only a few. Four meat packers control 90 percent of meat processing; eight firms control half (3.5 billion fowl) of the poultry industry.[3] Some 2 percent of all private corporations now control 90 percent of the agrichemical and feed-grain industries, and have a monopoly over 90 percent of the cattle, hog, and poultry industries.

The World's Top 12 Agribusinesses

United States	Philip Morris
United States	Cargill
Switzerland	Nestlé
UK/Netherlands	Unilever
United States	Pepsico
United States	Coca-Cola
United States	ConAgra
United States	RJR Nabisco
United Kingdom	Grand Metropolitan
Australia	Elder IKL
United States	Anheuser Busch
France	BSN Group

Source: PennAg Journal April 1997

The connection between the petrochemical-food and the biomedical-pharmaceutical industrial complex is yet another irony of the times. The former industry profits from selling agrichemical poisons, and the latter profits from treating a populace sickened, in part, by the food it eats. Agricultural ethicist Professor Martha Crouch contends,

The Rotten Roots of Agribusiness

"Agriculture cannot be sustainable if the primary purpose of growing food is to make a profit. Most food production is dominated by agribusiness, where profit is the main product and food is the means to get that profit."[4]

The World's Largest Meat Companies

The following list comprises a ranking of the 15 largest meat and poultry companies in the world ranked on the basis of annual sales converted into U.S. dollars. The parenthetical ranking of U.S. firms is the rank of that company in *Meat & Poultry*'s 1991 Top 100.

Rank	Rank	Company-Headquarters City	Annual Sales in U.S.$ (billions)
1.	(1)	ConAgra, Inc. - Omaha, Neb	12,500
2.	(2)	IBP, Inc. - Dakota City, Neb	10,388
3.	(3)	Cargill, Inc. - Minneapolis, Minn	5,800*
4.		Nippon Meat Packers, Inc. - Osaka, Japan	5,195
5.		Hillsdown Holdings Plc. - London, England	4,000+
6.	(4)	Tyson Foods, Inc. - Springdale, Ark	3,922
7.	(5)	Sara Lee Meat Group - Memphis, Tenn	3,000
8.		Itoham Foods, Inc. - Kobe City, Japan	2,986
9.	(6)	Geo. A. Hormel & Co., Inc. - Austin, Minn	2,836
10.	(7)	Oscar Mayer Foods - Madison, Wis.	2,500
11.		Union International Pic.- London, England	2,000
12.		Prima Meat Packers, Ltd. - Tokyo, Japan	1,987
13.	(8)	John Morrell & Co., Inc. - Cincinnati, Ohio	1,834
14.		The Sadia Group - Sao Paulo, Brazil	1,834
15.		Zenchiku Co., Ltd. - Tokyo, Japan	1,767

*red meat only   +estimate

Source: Meat & Poultry. April 1992.

It is inaccurate to blame agribusiness entirely for the multitude of problems that the profit motive has brought upon our food production system. Still, we need changes at the very roots of the system, from farm and field to farm policy and public support. The primary beneficiaries of today's food production system are the agribusiness and food industry conglomerates and the petrochemical-pharmaceutical industrial complex. The latter is now investing heavily in agricultural biotechnology, which promises further monopolistic control of the food production system and increased costs and dependence for the farming sector.

Farmers often have no other choice than to become corporate contract growers, taking whatever fixed price is offered. Family farms, which once sold chickens independently to processors on the open market some thirty years ago, today act exclusively as contract growers. This means the farmer contracts with a company to provide his labor and a facility to raise company chickens, on the company's feed, and to its specifications. Often this setup requires enormous capital outlay by the farmer to buy the necessary equipment for the intensive confinement systems. The same development is now occurring within the pork business.

This monopoly of the livestock industry allows corporations to establish larger livestock factories. In turn, this results in centralization of slaughter and processing facilities that causes loss of local jobs and markets in other areas. The direct and indirect costs to consumers of agribusiness monopolies therefore extends all the way to state unemployment insurance costs.

It is not a coincidence that Cargill and ConAgra—two of the largest agribusiness corporate monopolies in the world—combine grain trading and cattle feeding. The public is unaware that while livestock feed producers hardly make ends meet, these agribusiness monopolists enjoy fat public subsidies from livestock feed costs. (See the following sections in this chapter on government subsidies: *Government Subsidies and Ecological Bankruptcy* and *The Commodity Crop Treadmill*.)

Prices at the grocery store do not reflect these subsidies in a fair way. Smaller farmers cannot compete when the market prices for meat and other animal products are relatively low in relation to their own costs of production. Corporations have the advantage of high volume, and food prices will decline any time there is overproduction. Agribusiness corporations manipulate market prices through a variety of strategies that according to recent congressional investigations have included illegal price-fixing cartels; the corporations have essentially decided among themselves what they will pay farmers for their goods.

Corporations can sustain some net loss in the meat sector because they have diversified interests in other sectors of the food industry. This ability to take short-term losses in a particular area of the food industry serves to push small-scale, specialized corporations and independent farmers out of business. For example, all across America, supermarkets sell out-of-state (and out of country) produce that in turn puts local farmers out of business.

The food monopolists also exert control over the work force. Low wages, union-busting, and limited, if any, worker compensation are all scandalous realities in the meat- and poultry-packing sectors. Poultry processing is ranked as one of the country's most dangerous industries with an injury and illness incidence nearly twice that of coal mining and construction. Meat packers also suffer injuries in the workplace at about ten times the national average. Primary damage is to nerves and tendons as a result of repetitive motion injuries.

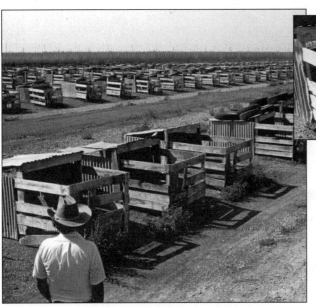

Photo: Michael W. Fox

Increasing the size of the operation to increase productivity and revenue, the less individual care animals receive. Calves in crates on dairy factory farms are being raised to replace spent cows.

The Cost of Industrialized Farming

The industrialized intensification of agriculture results in a host of environmental, economic, and social costs. These costs far outweigh the purported social benefit of a cheap and plentiful supply of food. Agribusiness (agri-bigness) has all but destroyed "agri-culture." At the

The Big Business of Agriculture

♦ Animal products contribute about 75 percent of the protein and one-third of the food energy in the American diet.

♦ Consumers spend around $230 billion annually on meat, poultry, eggs, and dairy products.

♦ Current annual value of the production, sale and processing of all food and fiber is around $700 billion, which amounts to 17 percent of the Gross National Product.

♦ In 1990, cattle and calves were the number-one farm product in eighteen states.

♦ Of the nearly $170 billion in agricultural cash receipts for that year, livestock and related products accounted for 52.7 percent or $89.6 billion, while crops brought in $80.4 billion.

♦ Concentration has meant an 85 percent decline in the number of pig farms since 1950.

♦ Three poultry companies now process nearly 40 percent of all broiler chickens.

♦ Over a million farms and ranches raise young beef cattle, yet only four companies process 60 percent of them.

♦ Concentration results in increased food transportation, handling, and marketing costs.

♦ The 1990 energy bill for marketing foods from United States farms was $16.5 billion,

♦ And inter-city transportation by truck and rail was nearly $20 billion.

turn of the century, agriculture employed 38 percent of the U.S. work force. Today, only about 2 percent of the population works in agriculture. Most of the farmland from those farmers who went out of business have been merged into larger holdings.[5] This shows a clear and steady trend toward corporate mega-farms. According to USDA predictions, the 50,000 largest farms in the United States will account for 75 percent of agricultural production by the year 2000.

The message to family farmers is "get big or get out." A generation ago a typical six hundred-acre farm would support more than one family, often with multiple generations. Now, because of agribusiness changes in market structure and the financial choke hold it places on farmers, it can now only support one generation. Sons and daughters must find employment elsewhere, or risk falling into the same financial trap.

There is another irony contained in the 1992 census report. The way farmers farm has been a major factor in the decline in farm residents. Agrichemicals and farm machinery such as huge tractors and combine harvesters increase agricultural productivity, which results in cycles of overproduction. In turn, this forces smaller farms to specialize, expand, or liquidate. The demise of smaller farms then affects the overall well-being of rural areas. With fewer farms, there is less need for support businesses in the towns of rural America. Many small communities have become veritable ghost towns with boarded-up store fronts and declining populations. Ultimately, this disintegration of rural communities fuels rising urban immigration, unemployment, crime, and poverty.

The technologies that result in more specialization, more production costs, and less local farming activity, are not suitable for a sustainable agriculture. The end result of this system of high-capital technological food production is the death of the family farm and rural communities. The disintegration of the rural community can cause even more profound changes in our society. Many great empires over the past seven thousand years have collapsed in large part because of nonsustainable agricultural practices.[6] Some say this will never happen to our industrial society because the technocracy knows best. So far technocracy certainly has not proven to have all the answers. Indeed, in many cases we can argue that science and technology, especially agricultural biotechnology, is extinguishing whatever potential remains for a sustainable and equitable agriculture.

Agrichemicals and Pesticides

Each year, American farmers use more than two hundred million pounds of pesticides, four hundred-fifty million pounds of herbicides, and forty million tons of chemical fertilizers on croplands. Corn, soybeans, wheat, and cotton receive over 90 percent of all pesticides used.

Since the turn of the century, the use of fertilizers and chemicals in farming has been questioned. In 1908 the first Annual Report of the Texas Commissioner of Agriculture stated, "There is absolutely no hope for the farmer so long as he depends utterly on dosing his starving land year after year with commercial fertilizers instead of building it up by stock raising and proper crop rotation."

Today, some ninety years later, the debate continues. Even with the increase in pesticide use, crop loss due to pests still increased 20 percent from mid-century levels, according to David Pimental, a Cornell University professor of entomology. And even though organic farming and integrated pest management (that includes breeding and distributing beneficial insects to control "pesky" ones) have shown to be viable, agribusiness relentlessly continues to use pesticides, despite the additional fact that many chemicals take hundreds of years to degrade.[7]

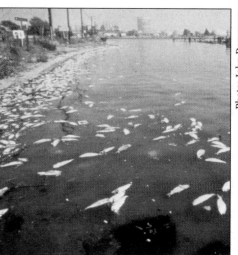

Fish kill in lake from agricultural runoff.

The pesticide industry has long denied that its products can cause cancer. However, exposure to agrichemicals weakens the immune system by suppressing the activity of white blood cells—T-helper cells and B cells that produce antibodies. In turn, this increases susceptibility to infectious diseases. Residues of pesticides, like DDT, chlordane, and industrial pollutants like dioxins and PCBs (polychlorinated biphenyls), are especially evident in animal fat. These chemicals and heavy metals, like mercury, which is common in fish, and cadmium, can cause the immune system to become hyperactive, resulting in autoimmune disorders such as thyroid disease and lupus when immune cells start attacking the body's own healthy tissue. Some pesticides, in combination with other chemicals like PCBs, become even more lethal, a phenomenon called "synergism."

These agrichemicals and industrial pollutants in our food and water (including plastic food wrapping and containers, and lacquer-coated food cans) have other disturbing physiological effects. Agrichemicals and industrial pollutants are hormone disrupters, and some mimic estrogen, the female sex hormone, and thus play a role in the development of endometriosis and estrogen-linked cancers, especially of the breast. Other agrichemicals block or otherwise disrupt normal hormonal functions, affecting growth, sexual development, fertility, mental development, and learning ability.[8]

Harmful effects of agrichemicals and industrial pollution are also evident in wildlife populations, putting some species at great risk of extinction. The impact on aquatic and terrestrial wildlife is so devastating that conventional agriculture has created poisoned wastelands. In spite of the evident risks of pesticides, a 1996 report released by the Environmental Protection Agency, "Pesticide Use in Agriculture," showed that farmers' use of pesticides reached record highs in 1994 and 1995. Farmers spent $10.4 billion in 1995 on these agrichemicals.

The annual revenue of the U.S. food industry totals more than $360 billion, and agrichemical sales are now almost $7 billion a year. So there was much to fear if the public had panicked following the June 1993 release of a long overdue study[9] on the risks of agrichemicals to children. The study states:

> **There should be a presumption of greater toxicity to infants and children. In such cases, the National Academy of Sciences panel called for exposure standards ten times more stringent than would normally be applied.[10]**

The Clinton administration moved quickly to quell public concern by calling on the United States Department of Agriculture (USDA), the Environmental Protection Agency (EPA), and the Federal Food and Drug Administration (FDA), to work together (a first indeed) on this serious issue. Unfortunately, it is already too little and too late for millions of children. Particularly disturbing in this report is the evidence of the continuing presence of various pesticides in human breast milk.

In addition, I found particularly dubious, ethically and scientifically, the study's recommendation to conduct more tests on young rodents to determine how they react to chemicals compared to mature animals .

More than forty-five thousand different pesticides, formulated from fourteen hundred active ingredients, find their way onto the American market. Rigorous toxicity evaluation is incomplete for most of these active ingredients. In 1984 there were no safety data—at all—for 37 percent of the active ingredients in common use.[11] Manufacturers market new pesticides every year, and place the burden of proof of safety evaluation on the government, all at taxpayers' expense. The EPA is so far behind on its safety testing schedule that it might *never* meet its legislated responsibilities.

Dependence on chemical fertilizers and pesticides is so pervasive in its effect that it fouls the entire food chain, the very center of the ecological web of life. It is indeed unfortunate that mainstream agriculture chose to adopt this dependence on a finite petrochemical resource—we now have an agriculture that is inherently not sustainable, because we will eventually run out of fossil fuels. Since farmers use chemicals in place of animal—and human—manure, animals cease to be an integrated component of natural farming. Today, animals live in feedlots and confinement buildings rather than on the land. The chain is broken.

Farmers' Health Hazards

The health hazards to farmers who use agrichemicals are at last being recognized and researched. "Farmers have higher than normal rates of leukemia, multiple myeloma, non-Hodgkins lymphoma and cancers of the brain, prostate, stomach, skin and lip," says Charles Lynch, M.D., of the University of Iowa College of Medicine, Iowa City. "Chronic diseases like asthma, neurologic and kidney disease also may be related to agricultural exposures."[12] According to studies in the United Kingdom, farmers who have frequent exposure to agrichemicals have been found to have memory deficits, slower reaction times, and are more prone to psychiatric disorders. In addition, male sperm counts among farm workers have declined nearly 50 percent in the past two generations. It seems that farmers and farm workers are latter-day miners' canaries, if not the guinea pigs, for biomedical research.

A September 1992 National Cancer Institute study also confirmed that farmers have elevated risks of several forms of cancer. Over-exposure to pesticides is one suspected cause, along with fertilizer in drinking water, fuels and oils, and fumigants, to which farmers are far more exposed than those not involved in agriculture.[13]

Entomology professor David Pimental, points out that there has been a 33 percent increase in the use of increasingly potent pesticides since the 1940s. However, crop losses to fungi, weeds, and insects have actually increased from around 31 percent in the 1940s to today's average of 37 percent. Pimental estimates that farmers can reduce their use of agrichemicals by half simply by employing biological pest control methods, such as releasing ladybugs to control green flies, and using crop rotation. Contrary to agribusiness claims, food prices would not skyrocket. Instead prices would increase by less than 1 percent. To offset this "price increase," Pimental calculates that the country will save up to $10 billion per year in decreased costs of pesticide regulation, increased quality of our drinking water and fish stocks, and decreased health care costs for the tens-of-thousands of people who suffer from pesticide poisoning.[14]

Growers use a tremendous amount of toxic chemicals on the crops they grow for livestock feed. When the animals eat the feed, these chemicals accumulate in their tissues.[15] Beef contains the highest concentration of herbicides of any food and ranks third of all foods in insecticide contamination. Meat contains approximately fourteen times more pesticides than plants.[16] About 95 percent of the toxic chemicals found in our diet come from eggs, dairy products, fish, and meat. Toxins are easily stored in fat, and each step up on the food chain consumes more toxins. Fish, in particular, have long food chains. Even avoiding eating fish to limit exposure to toxins might not be possible, since about one third of the world's catch of fish is fed to livestock.[17]

According to Pimental, "Of more than six hundred pesticides now in use, the National Residue Program tests for only forty-one that are determined to be of public health concern. The meat is generally sold and consumed before the test results are available."[18] Worldwide, these chemicals account for some twenty thousand deaths and one million illnesses per year.[19]

The good news is that the public strongly opposes the continued use of pesticides. A public survey conducted in 1993 by the consumer advocacy organization, Public Voice for Food and Health Policy, reveals the following:

♦ 71 percent of Americans feel a great concern about pesticides and fertilizers in drinking water.

♦ 60 percent of Americans believe it is very important for farmers to farm organically, using chemicals only as a last resort.

♦ 84 percent think the government should be actively encouraging farmers to use fewer chemicals and pesticides.

♦ 71 percent want to see stores stock more "low-chemical foods."

♦ 86 percent believe people have the right to know how many chemicals the farmers and processors are using on foods sold at the supermarket.

♦ Half strongly agree that they would accept "ugly looking" fruit if they knew that the fruit was grown with fewer pesticides.[20]

If the results of this survey are true, then why has the government ignored the public's will? Whose interests are more important—the chemical agribusiness industry or the consumer?

Pesticides and the Cancer Threat

Five potential cancer-causing herbicides commonly used by farmers in the Midwest and Chesapeake Bay region are seeping into soil, rivers, and streams and appearing in tap water.[21] More than fourteen million people are at risk. Midwest farmers use some 150 million pounds of herbicides every year, particularly on corn and soybeans raised to feed farm animals. Herbicides identified include Alachlor (marketed under the trade name Lasso), Metolachlor, Atrazine, Cyanazine, and Simazine.

In the 1950s and 1960s, five chlorinated compounds—unlike other pesticides in that they are not readily broken down—were widely used by agriculture. These compounds were: Dichlorodiphenyltrichloroethane (DDT), Dieldrin, Chlordane, Mirex, and Heptachior, all of which were banned in the 1970s by the EPA. These five pesticides are, and will be, found in fish for decades due to agricultural runoff into lakes, rivers, and oceans.

The EPA believes that the dietary risk from these banned pesticides is low in most foods.[22] But as we now know there is a high potential for these persistent pesticides to concentrate over time in fish.

However, the mounting evidence against pesticides should motivate farmers to take immediate action to drastically reduce herbicide use and adopt well-tested alternative methods of weed control. As North Dakota organic grain grower Fred Kirschenmann says, "Once we add in the social and environmental costs, we'll find out just how expensive our current agricultural system is. But we can change it, if we want to."[23]

In addition to agribusiness' impact on our deadly diets, industrial pollution—especially the chemical dioxin from incinerated industrial waste, chemical plants, and paper mills—spreads by wind and rain and eventually enters the food chain. Dioxin is one of the most toxic of all chemicals. An EPA draft released in September 1994 entitled, "Dioxin Reassessment," found dioxin in various foods at levels that could cause cancer. Dioxin is implicated in damaging our immune and reproductive systems, and can cause developmental and hormone-regulation disorders in humans and other animals. According to this EPA report:

♦ Beef accounts for more than one-third of the estimated daily exposure to dioxin-like compounds;

♦ Dairy products account for 24.1 percent;

♦ Milk accounts for 17.6 percent;

♦ Chicken and pork hover around 12 percent;

♦ Fish accounts for 7.8 percent;

♦ Eggs account for 4.1 percent.

Because dioxins concentrate primarily in animal fat and milk, including human breast milk, fruits and vegetables are less of a consumer risk. Alarmingly, high dioxin levels in a mother's milk are likely if nursing mothers consume a lot of animal fat and protein.[24]

Free-ranging cattle accumulate dioxin in their body fat because they eat contaminated vegetation. They also may ingest dioxins from eating contaminated soil. On arid and overgrazed ranges late in the grazing season this soil can be as much as 18 percent of the animals' diet because there is nothing else to eat.

Animal fat and fish meals high in dioxins are ground up at the rendering plant in order to make livestock feed and pet food. This food source most likely leads to further concentration of this poisonous group of chemicals to the detriment of livestock, consumers, and pets.

In order to cut feed costs, farmers give their cattle byproducts such as brewer's grains, tomato and citrus pulp. However, these otherwise nutritious food-industry wastes contain pesticide residues and toxic molds such as aflatoxin. They present a consumer risk because poisons such as aflatoxin concentrate in animal fat, butter fat, and egg yolk.

Bioaccumulation is when toxic chemicals concentrate as they travel higher up the food chain with farm animals in the middle, and humans at the top. Farm animals concentrate industrial chemical pollutants in their bodies. These pass on to consumers in the milk, eggs, meat, liver, and other organs. Because animals concentrate far more hazardous chemicals in their tissues than most plants, a shift toward a more plant-based diet is a wise consumer response.

Government Inspectors and Contaminated Food

It took until January 31, 1995, for the USDA to announce a plan to improve the grossly inadequate visual inspection system for meat. The traditional system failed, causing almost five million cases of illness and more than four thousand deaths associated with contaminated or diseased meat and poultry products each year. This system was referred to

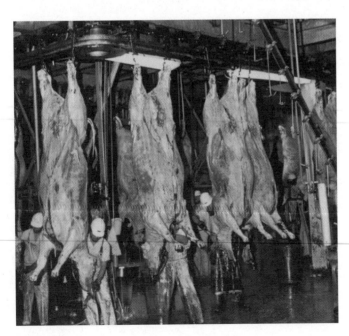

High speed processing inevitably leads to meat contamination from harmful bacteria.

as "organoleptic" inspection, which meant the government inspector had only a few seconds to look at a carcass as it passed on a conveyor moving at such a fast rate that inspectors suffered from "line fatigue."

Through a hidden camera, an employee of a South Dakota slaughterhouse managed to video tape for CBS TV's "48 Hours" how three hundred employees processed an average of fifty cows per hour with only four USDA inspectors on hand. The tape showed the meat cutters violating USDA rules when taking dangerous shortcuts cleaning up abscess fluids from a piece of beef. One long-time USDA veterinarian said, "I can say from my experience of nine years and in talking to other food inspectors around the country, this probably goes on on a daily basis."[25]

One in every three broiler chickens are contaminated with harmful bacteria due in part to inadequate inspection.

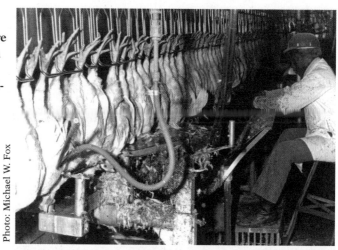

Photo: Michael W. Fox

The USDA does not require that poultry processors check for *Salmonella* bacteria, even though The Center for Science in the Public Interest reports that 25 percent of all chickens sold in the United States carry the *Salmonella* bacteria. A 1978 USDA regulation accepts a "chill tank" bath for carcasses as a preventative measure. This dip, known as "fecal soup," has been compared to a rinse in the toilet.[26] The new USDA plan includes rinsing carcasses in a microbicidal wash, stricter meat-handling rules, plus daily random sample tests for *Salmonella*. It is important to note that the food industry in general opposes the new food-handling regulations because of added costs and slowdown in the rate of processing.

Government food safety regulators speak enthusiastically about their scientifically based system called "Hazard Analysis and Critical Control Point" (HACCUP, pronounced "hassup"). This is a process that will ostensibly identify where microbial hazards are most likely to be present so they can institute preventive steps. The problem with this new system is that it still ignores the reality that potentially harmful bacteria are everywhere. The six billion poultry and one hundred twenty-five million livestock carcasses slaughtered each year are grown on factory farms that serve as incubators and breeding grounds for hazardous microbes. Potentially harmful bacteria contaminate up to one in every three broiler chickens.

The number of people becoming sick, chronically ill, and even dying from foodborne diseases after consuming meat, eggs, or dairy products is so considerable that we should consider these diseases as the *new* plagues brought on by the industrialization of animal agriculture. According to the Family Food Protection Act of 1995, Section 2: "[M]eat and meat food products, and poultry and poultry products, contaminated with pathogenic bacteria are a leading cause of foodborne illness."[27]

Government scientist, Dr. Jean Buzby, collated these disturbing findings about foodborne illnesses in 1993:

- Foodborne *Salmonella* cases numbered 696,000 to 3,840,000 and resulted in 696 to 3,840 deaths in the United States;

- Foodborne *Campylobacter* cases numbered 1,418,494 to 1,805,356 and resulted in 110 to 511 deaths;

- Foodborne *E. coli* 0157:H7 cases numbered 8,000 to 16,000 and resulted in 160 to 400 deaths;

- Foodborne *Lysteria monocytogenes* cases numbered 1,526 to 1,767 and resulted in 377 to 475 deaths.

Dr. Buzby estimates a total number of foodborne disease cases for the four pathogens of 3,390,875 to 6,600,940, resulting in 1,644 to 5,730 deaths in the United States.[28]

Medical costs and lost productivity for the four pathogens resulting from foodborne illness ranged from $1.73 billion to $5.3 billion. Foodborne *C. jejuni*-induced Guillain-Barré syndrome (GBS), causes an additional $179 million to $902 million in losses, with total foodborne illness losses of $1.9 billion to $6.2 billion.

The *E. coli* 0157:H7 strain, found in cattle fecal matter (which often contaminates meat), produces a toxin that causes human kidney failure. This harmful bacterium was first identified in 1982, and is the cause of at least fifty-five outbreaks in the United States. Unbelievably, only thirty-one states currently require reporting of this infection.

The shocking outbreaks of *E. coli* 0157:H7 food poisoning and death from contaminated meat prompted the U.S. government to propose irradiation as the right solution. However, irradiation is no substitute for improved livestock and poultry care and slaughter procedures.

Numerous conditions contribute to bacterial proliferation and contamination. These include overcrowding and poor sanitation on farm and feedlot; stress from inhumane handling and transportation; contaminated feed from fish meal and rendered offal or "animal tankage"; high-speed processing; and poor slaughterhouse sanitation.

The USDA's Animal and Plant Health Inspection Service (APHIS) noted that the number of *E. coli* 0157:H7 organisms "are shown to increase in the gastrointestinal tracts of stressed and starved animals and birds." Other studies find that stress during transportation of animals from the farm to slaughter increases the spreading of *Salmonella*. Specifically, slaughter calves that spent more than twelve hours in transit or holding had an incidence of *Salmonella* infection about 40 percent higher than calves slaughtered within twelve hours of leaving the farm.[29]

Following public outcry over *E. coli* food safety problems, the Food Safety Inspection Service (FSIS) said that it would test meat for bacterial contamination. According to Dr. Lyle P. Vogel, who favors the "hassup" system, to do this effectively would cost over $15 billion a year, adding approximately $2.17 to the cost of each pound of ground beef.[30]

Government Subsidies and Ecological Bankruptcy

The publicly subsidized grazing program in the United States is a serious hidden cost to consumers, and a highly controversial issue. Ranchers in the Western states pay close to $2 per month for each unit of public land capable of sustaining one cow, one horse, or five sheep. The land is assessed at how many cattle it can support, each animal being one "unit" and the grazing fee being due every month. Hence the grazing fee is per "animal unit month." The U.S. Government Accounting Office (GAO) states that this paltry fee does not cover government costs of administration and rangeland management. Livestock grazing at ridiculously cheap rents now takes place on 44 percent of the public land base in the United States, excluding Alaska.

Some 265 million acres of federal lands are involved in this subsidized grazing program. Yet, according to the USDA, only 2 percent of the cattle and sheep produced annually come off these lands. That such a relatively small percentage of animals should cause so much ecological harm is pause for concern. Of the public rangelands administered by the United States Forest Service and Bureau of Land Management, some 70 percent of this land is in unacceptable condition due to overgrazing, according to the USDA. This has resulted in some 10 percent of the arid West being turned into desert. Yet, taxpayers spend upwards of $100 million a year to subsidize ranchers' use and abuse of these public lands.

The National Cattlemen's Association and other livestock industry organizations have effectively blocked attempts by Congress to legislate an increase in grazing fees, which can be as low as $1.61 a unit, with an average around $1.92 per unit. New legislation would have increased the grazing fees by nearly four times to about $5.36 per unit. The financial resources of some very wealthy corporations helped to effectively crush this long overdue legislation. Wealthy corporations that benefit from a below-cost federal grazing program fund the Washington D.C. livestock industry lobbyists.

Ironically, outmoded grazing laws made in the nineteenth century to help small ranching operations on public lands now enable giant corporations to make billions of dollars at taxpayers' expense. For example, the National Wildlife Federation, in a 1992 study of corporate exploitation of public lands, found that three out-of-state companies paid the federal government a mere $235,000 to let their livestock graze on 2.4 million acres of public land in southeast Oregon. Ninety percent of that land is in unsatisfactory condition, according to government studies. A GAO report released in April 1993 on cattle and sheep grazing on public lands controlled by the United States Forest Service revealed a similar picture.

An April 1992 review by the Bureau of Land Management and Forest Service found that in 1990 alone, permit fees collected from ranchers fell $52 million short of covering the costs of the grazing programs. A mere 6 percent of those holding grazing permits to use Forest

Service land control almost half of the animals allowed to graze on range managed by this agency. Some of the largest grazing allotments belong to the Federal Mutual Insurance Company, the Church Universal and Triumphant of Livingston, Montana, and the Hunt Oil Company of Dallas, Texas.

Abuse of public lands results in overgrazing. These cattle starved to death on a degraded range.

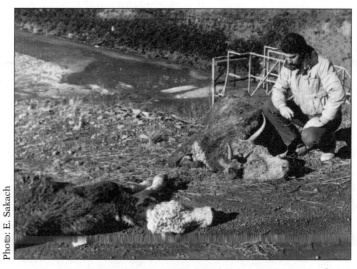

Photo: E. Sakach

A common practice in New Mexico is for ranchers to sublease the subsidized public lands they control. They sublet the land at market value to other ranchers anywhere from twice to ten times what they pay the federal government, and simply pocket the difference. Ranchers who sublease their public lands now pay the government a paltry $1.61 per animal unit month and collect on average $7 in the open market. On one site in southeastern New Mexico, auctioned forage recently sold for as much as $16.38 per animal unit month.[31]

Currently the battle over ranchers' rights to use public lands for grazing versus government attempts to enforce compliance with environmentally protective range management directives is close to becoming an insurrection. Ranchers are uniting, and are demanding home rule, and carte blanche use of public lands. "Folks are taking the law into their own hands," said Jim Nelson, an outspoken career government official who supervises the Toiyabe and Humboldt National Forests in Nevada. "We're going to have anarchy and chaos in eastern Nevada," he told the press. "We can't protect the resource because we are afraid our employees will be shot," added Ann Morgan, Nevada state director of the Bureau of Land Management (BLM). "It's not worth that."[32]

Catering primarily to agribusiness interests, Federal Farm Bill budget priorities have changed little over the past two decades. Within the staggering USDA appropriation of $82.6 billion for fiscal year 1992, only a mere $125 million was appropriated for the Agricultural Conservation Program designed to protect wildlife habitat and prevent erosion.[33] The budget to develop new methods to kill livestock predators (like improved poison-bait delivery systems) and crop pests was $9.5 million, while the entire Sustainable Agriculture Research and Education program (SARE) was given a paltry $6.75 million. The USDA's special grants totaling $447,000 were for beef carcass evaluation and identification of fat content. Of that amount, $200,000 went for beef producers' marketing enhancement through carcass improvement, which is aimed at reducing fat content. This use of public money is not in synch with the vision of a cost-effective and efficient food production system.

Each year in the United States, an area the size of Connecticut is lost to topsoil erosion; 85 percent of this erosion is linked to livestock production. Two hundred years ago, American topsoil measured an average of twenty-one inches. Today, only six inches remain. We have lost over one-third of the topsoil of United States cropland in just one hundred years. There is no price tag yet on the estimated four to five billion tons of topsoil lost annually from erosion. Likewise, there is no price tag on the degradation of marginal lands and rangeland from overgrazing, and the loss of wildlife and natural biodiversity.

Unique ecosystems held under public trust and the legal authority of state and federal agencies are being irreparably harmed by agricultural practices that are in violation of the National Environmental Policy Act (NEPA). For example, individual state irrigation programs receive heavy subsidies. In Arizona, the government subsidizes water to operate huge dairy feedlots; California subsidizes the export of crops such as cotton, broccoli, fruits, and other agricultural commodities to other states and nations; and Florida subsidizes citrus groves and sugar cane fields. All of these state-subsidized programs are destroying state and federal wildlife preserves. The Florida Everglades are disappearing, and so are the mountain lakes, forests, and bright savannas of California.

We can calculate some costs such as the loss of topsoil and other natural resources, the demise of rural communities, public health and food safety, and farm animal diseases. But how do we reckon these costs along with the vast expenditures of public funds on farm commodity price supports and subsidies? These subsidies include expensive irrigation projects to provide cheap water, predator-control programs on public lands, and cheap grazing fees for cattle ranchers. The Carter administration Secretary of Agriculture, Bob Bergland, said it best: "If we assessed the true cost of grazing livestock on public lands, we would let it go back to wildlife."

Ironically, farm subsidy programs originally designed to help farmers now help those least in need. According to the United States Department of Agriculture, 30 percent of all subsidies went to farm operators earning $100,000 or more per year, approximately 4 percent of the entire farming population. Attempts by legislators to reform this public subsidization of agribusiness mega-farms and food industry conglomerates fail year after year, in part because of the financial generosity of the industry for campaign contributions at election time. Both the House and Senate Agriculture Committees consist of strong supporters of farm programs, who do not evaluate these programs critically. Political scientists describe this phenomenon as the committees being "captured" by the very industries they are regulating.

The Commodity Crop Treadmill

Most people do not know about—or understand—how the United States government's commodity crop program works. Many who do are outraged. It is a complex program that guarantees farmers a fixed price support for corn, soybeans or other commodity crops, and regulates how many acres of land the farmers can plant. Some years the government tells farmers to set aside a certain amount of acreage and pays them not to produce the designated commodity crop from these acres.

The net result is to maintain a high level of production nationwide, which generally results in a relatively low market price for the commodity producers. Low prices especially benefit the food-industry corporations because this in turn provides them with a public subsidy for the grains, livestock, and poultry feed they purchase.

Meanwhile, farmers' profits remain low, while consumer prices generally increase. Farmers who want to get off this commodity crop treadmill and stop ecologically unsound monocrop farming are unable to do so unless they give up their reliance on crop subsidies. Such an inflexible government system is not good for the land, for the farmers, or for the economy. It forces farmers to compete and expand their production rather than farm ecologically in ways suited to their region and climate.

In the 1996 Farm Bill, euphemistically called the "Freedom to Farm Bill," significant changes in commodity subsidy policies were made. Market prices are no longer supported and the government no longer tells farmers how much, what, or where to plant, since most are now contracted to large agribusiness companies anyway. Farmers still get subsidies, but there are no strings attached. Plans are to eliminate farm subsidies by 2002 so that we will have a "free market." However, in my opinion, subsidies should be continued to encourage farmers to shift to organic production methods.

But the cost to Americans cannot only be counted in dollars; it must also take into consideration the major damage caused to the environment. E. Goldsmith and N. Hildyard's landmark documentation in their book, *The Earth Report*, points out that over half of the United States' original natural wetlands have been lost primarily to agriculture.[34] Natural wetlands act as a sponge, absorbing heavy rains and thus preventing rivers from flooding. This is now a major problem especially in the Midwest where wetlands have been drained and converted for agriculture.

Forest fires are another national problem that the cattle industry may actually contribute to. Overgrazing of our forest lands contributes to forest fires that seem to get worse every year. In a natural forest, dry grasses and other vegetation burn after a lightning strike and kill off tree seedlings, leaving old trees standing that are fire resistant. Grazing cattle remove these grasses so there is no kindling to control the growth of saplings, which proliferate. So when lightning strikes, millions of small trees go up in flames, which leads to thousands of acres of devastated land. There are few fire-resistant trees left since most were clear-cut decades ago by the timber industry throughout most of the United States.

There exists the attitude that when nature's resources run out, technology will find the right answers. This is a pervasive flaw in industrial agriculture's thinking. Almost half the irrigated land in the United States is in regions where groundwater tables are being irreparably depleted. For example, the massive, Midwestern Ogallala Aquifer that extends from Nebraska to Texas supplies water to one-fifth of all irrigated crops in the United States. Spanning more than eight Midwestern states, this natural resource from the Ice Age may be gone within several decades because of modern agribusiness sucking it dry to grow grain for livestock feed.[35]

The rate of groundwater pumping in California's San Joaquin Valley now exceeds natural replenishment by an estimated one-half trillion gallons per year. When these finite groundwater reserves disappear, mega-farm owners will want to drain more lakes and divert more rivers for irrigation. The mega-farm owners will justify the ecological damage that will result by reasoning that it is an "unavoidable necessity." Over half of the total amount of water consumed in this country is used to irrigate land for raising livestock feed. Our diminishing supply of drinkable water is directly linked to meat consumption. Masanobu Fukuoka, founder of Japan's natural farming, observes:

> Man also makes crop disease and pest control indispensable by growing unhealthy crops. Agricultural technology creates the causes that produce disease and pest damage, then becomes adept at treating these. Scientific farming attempts to correct and improve on what it perceives as the shortcomings of nature through human effort. In contrast, when a problem arises, natural farming relentlessly pursues the causes and strives to correct and restrain human action.[36]

According to proponents of industrial agriculture, the fact that the urban populace has a cheap and plentiful supply of food outweighs all costs. They claim that the miracles of agricultural food technology—processing, marketing, and distribution—make it possible to feed millions of nonfarming city folk. However, consumers do not realize the long-term impact and great costs to future generations of this plentiful, cheap, meat-based food supply.

The Shrinking Genetic Pool

Another very real concern that affects everyone is the rapid disappearance of all but a few varieties of crop seed stock, and livestock and poultry breeds. This loss of genetic resources and diversity makes the agricultural system more inflexible and vulnerable to pests and dis-eases. Manufacturers can increase genetic diversity by creating new patented varieties of genetically engineered seeds and farm animals. However, this will do nothing to alleviate the loss of these basic genetic resources. Such resources are extremely valuable when farming prac-tices need adaptation because of epidemic disease, climatic, and other environmental changes.

The loss of genetic resources has become a major threat to biologi-cal diversity. Agribusiness propagates certain commercial and patented varieties. This usually excludes more genetically varied, often more dis-ease-resistant, and regionally adaptable strains and breeds. Livestock grazing is the primary reason for the elimination or endangerment of various plant species in North America. The ancestors of our modern cattle lived in wetter and greener ecosystems that were better able to withstand the abuse from grazing.[37]

Conservationists estimate that we have lost more than half the vari-eties of the world's twenty most important food crops that existed at the beginning of this century. These include corn, rice, wheat, potatoes, and bananas. Over the same period we have allowed 80 percent of the varieties of horticultural fruit crops in the United States to disappear. More than one-third of livestock and poultry breeds in the United States are rare or in decline, and half of the breeds in Europe that existed at the turn of the century are now extinct.[38] We must hope that the recently initiated Food and Agriculture Organization's Biodiversity Conservation Program to protect these vital genetic resources is not too little too late.

Corporate interests are lobbying to block any legislation to permit the labeling of genetically engineered food. Proper labeling would also show methods used to grow the food, such as organic, free range, and in what region or country it originated.

The only way to ensure a greener world and more healthful agricul-ture for future generations is to break free of the monopolistic control that agribusiness corporations have over agricultural markets. We can do this by supporting those markets where mega-corporations have lit-tle or no control. That includes our local farmers' markets, and organic and humane sustainable farmers and ranchers. We need a strong alliance between concerned consumers who share the view that we do not inherit the land, we borrow it from our children.

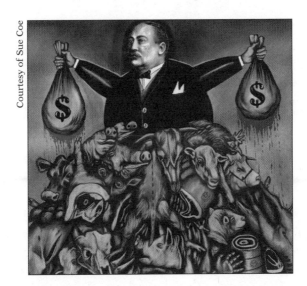

Courtesy of Sue Coe

Taxpayers Subsidize Agribusiness Advertising

Government promotional subsidies ostensibly help create more jobs in the United States via product advertising and marketing internationally. These subsidies have been considerable and benefit large multinational and transnational corporations. According to a detailed investigation in 1993 by the *Washington Post*, since 1986, more than $400 million has been given to United States companies for advertising.[39] Within the same ten years, an additional $600 million was simply given by the government to agribusiness corporations for generic advertisements promoting agricultural commodities ranging from beef to bourbon. These export marketing subsidies do not consider the companies' or producer associations size and annual profits. A sample list of USDA marketing promotion subsidies includes:

- ◆ Sunniest Growers: $66.6 million;
- ◆ Blue Diamond: $35.7 million;
- ◆ Dole: $15 million;
- ◆ Gallo Wine: $14.5 million;
- ◆ Tyson Foods: $11.1 million;
- ◆ Pillsbury: $8.7 million;
- ◆ Welch's: $5.1 million;
- ◆ M&M/Mars: $3.8 million.[40]

And the list goes on. Foreign firms received $78 million to encourage them to use U.S. suppliers of cotton and other U.S. agricultural commodities. According to the same *Washington Post* report, Congressman Peter H. Kostmayer (D-Pa), probably lost his re-election campaign when he called taxpayer-supported advertising "an especially egregious program."[41]

Some manufacturers, such as candy manufacturers, complain that they need such help because USDA price supports boost the cost of the milk, sugar, raisins, and peanuts they need. They claim they often have to pay double the world price of sugar.

All of this may be a bargaining chip for much-needed international reform in agricultural commodity pricing. Full-cost accounting and equitable world market pricing, coupled with supply-management, are necessary initiatives at this time. The final round of General Agreement on Trade and Tariffs (GATT) negotiations failed to make this an integral part of its final creation of the World Trade Organization (WTO).

The United States is competing with the European Economic Community (EEC) and both are weaving a socially unjust, inequitable food industry based on nonsustainable agriculture that is harming the environment, rural communities, and urban consumers. GATT and the WTO may bring about some reduction in competition, but they will most likely make the world an exclusive playing field of transnational corporations. It is, conveniently, illegal under WTO rules for countries to set up trade barriers to protect their own farmers from being undercut by domestic markets being flooded by "cheaper" imported agricultural commodities.

Under the 1996 Agricultural Export Enhancement program, hundreds of millions of dollars are being given out of the public coffers by the U.S. government, not to help farmers develop more productive methods of sustainable agriculture, but to multinational corporations like Cargill and Tyson Foods. The aim is to lower export costs to facilitate the sale of agricultural produce abroad and to encourage the adoption of U.S. agribusiness technology, seeds, fertilizers, farming methods, and hog and poultry factories in countries like Russia and China, as well as in Asia and South and Central America.

Many of these subsidized exports (which may be GATT illegal) will undercut the fair market price of indigenous farmers' produce. The net result will be the demise of rural communities and other sustainable and self-sufficient farming methods as industrial agriculture becomes global, doing to other countries what is being done to the farming communities of much of North America and western Europe. Because member countries cannot set up trade barriers and tariffs in order to protect their own farmers—which are not permissible under World Trade Organization's laws and conventions—other countries will also fall victim to agri-industrial imperialism. Even now, they are being coerced into the industrial mode of high-input, intensive crop and livestock production as their own farmers are forced to get big or to get out.

School Promotion of Agribusiness Interests

With taxpayers' money via government subsidies, agribusiness influences American youth through school programs. Government funds are being used to promote the meat industry directly in the public school system under the guise of "educational materials." For example, "Ag in the Classroom" is a program that received over $200,000 in taxpayer dollars for 1997 largely to promote animal agribusiness to school children.

The pork industry is even targeting preschoolers with a kit of materials distributed to child-care centers and preschools as part of its "Youth Initiative" to promote the consumption of pigs. The kit is a revision of one developed by the beef industry and is financed with check-off funds, which are tax-exempt moneys used for product promotion and other purposes.

With private funding, the National Dairy Council has formed a "nutrition education partnership" with one of the nation's largest day care providers. And five mobile "dairy classrooms," sponsored by the Dairy Council of California, spread the dairy industry's message of milk consumption to seven hundred thousand school kids every year.

Critical thinking is essential in the classroom, yet attempts to present children with views differing from those of agribusiness are often blocked. Children must have access to all legitimate views about diet and how their food is produced if they are to develop the ability to make informed consumer decisions.

Agribusiness Protecting the Status Quo

Control of information about agribusiness practices and interests has influenced controversial legislation that is now in place in several states such as Texas and Iowa. This new legislation makes it a felony to photograph or video tape livestock or poultry operations. The purpose of this legislation is to prevent the documentation of the intensive and often cruel conditions under which most food animals live. By doing this, state and federal legislators are endeavoring to isolate animal agriculture from public censure and accountability. Several states have also put in place what is called the "Food Disparagement Act," which essentially makes any individual subject to litigation if he or she says anything negative and unsubstantiated in public about milk from cows injected with recombinant bovine growth hormone, about pork from factory farmed pigs, or about eggs from poultry factory farms. Even though such legislation is in clear violation of the Constitution's First Amendment (freedom of speech) it illustrates how powerful the agribusiness food industry has become, and to what extremes it will go to maintain business interests.

Opposition to informed public concern over how the land and farm animals are being treated is intensifying. In the spring of 1997, several members of Congress reintroduced a so-called "FDA Reform" bill, HR 1411. Specifically, "national labeling uniformity" provisions in "Section 28" of this proposed "Drug and Biological Products Modernization Act of 1997" will make it nearly impossible for consumers to know whether food has been genetically engineered or not, whether toxic pesticides and other carcinogenic residues remain on food products, and whether cosmetics have been produced in an animal "cruelty-free" manner. The bill, according to Ronnie Cummins, director of the Pure Food Campaign, would outlaw local and state "rBGH-free" labeling and advertising and make it all but impossible to require mandatory labeling of genetically engineered foods and crops. Section 28 basically prevents states or local legislative bodies from initiating labeling laws relating to food safety, genetically engineered foods, or "cruelty-free" cosmetics.

Cummins and other critics point out that the FDA Reform bill appears to be yet another manifestation of the new global economic order under the GATT agreements. If passed, local, state, and national laws in regard to food safety, genetic engineering, pesticides, and disclosure of food or cosmetic production methods will be eliminated or weakened in order to facilitate the rapid development and monopolization of global markets by giant transnational corporations—in this case multinational chemical, factory farm, biotechnology, pharmaceutical, and cosmetics firms. This type of anti-consumer legislation becomes necessary for the industry as consumer alarm intensifies over genetic engineering, factory farming, food safety, cloning, and animal cruelty.

Amazingly, this legislation comes at a time when consumers are awakening to the dangers in their environment. A 1997 poll conducted by agribusiness multinational corporation, Novartis, found that 93 percent of American consumers demand mandatory labeling of genetically engineered foods, and 54 percent desire organic production methods. Other similar polls have found 80 percent of consumers expressing concern about food safety and pesticide residues, with 66 percent opposed to the cloning of animals. As the success of cruelty-free cosmetics and dolphin-safe tuna have shown, consumer outcries cannot be stifled for long.

Consumers are realizing that corporate directors of the multinational agribusiness corporations do not usually include in their decision making ethical, moral, environmental, and animal welfare concerns. A market-driven, conventional, industrial agriculture is the antithesis of a democratic, consumer-farmer integrated eco-agriculture. *All* people should have a say in how we raise and treat our food and in how we treat the land and animals.

Wanted: Government Support

With enough organizations and individuals placing pressure on the government and its politicians, there is hope. The urgent need to make U.S. agriculture more sustainable has resulted in marginally better funding from the government. Funding is still in the "millions," instead of in the "billions" where it should be. By 1995 appropriations for the Sustainable Agriculture Research and Education (SARE) program, including extension programs in sustainable agriculture (often referred to as Chapter 3 programs) and the Agriculture in Concert With Environment (ACE) program, was about $12 million.

In 1996 the administration secured $1.2 million for the Agricultural Technology and Transfer for Rural Areas (ATTRA) program. Authorized by the Farm Bill, ATTRA was first funded in 1987. It serves the entire nation with specialists who provide farmers and others with sustainable agriculture information, research results, and practical information. There is no other source of readily available information covering such a wide scope of sustainable agriculture topics. In 1994 ATTRA serviced more than twelve thousand inquiries from farmers and other interested people. The increased funding for fiscal year 1996 will allow ATTRA to meet informational requests and to pursue other important projects. Some of their projects include building a database and sharing resources and results concerning on-farm and community-based, value-added (such as goods that are baked or cured), and market development activities.

By 1995 the total budget for all USDA programs was almost $62 billion. The important Conservation Reserve Program, where highly erodible lands remain out of production and set aside for wildlife habitat, cost $1,859,000 in 1995. The Natural Resources Conservation Service received $4,210,000 in 1995. They are responsible for conservation operations, the wetlands reserve program, forest management, watershed, and flood prevention operations.

The Food and Safety Inspection Service (FSIS) received an increase in funding to $678 million in 1995. This is in response to the increasing incidence of food poisoning from contaminated meat and poultry. However, it is unlikely that no matter how much public money is given out to the FSIS, the problem of foodborne diseases will not diminish or be contained if agribusiness continues "business as usual." The solutions lie in people eating fewer foods of animal origin and in the abolition of factory farms and feedlots.

Government funding of the Cooperative State Research, Education, and Extension Service to facilitate sustainable agriculture under the Clinton administration has been small but has increased over the years, with $9.5 million being allotted in the 1996 budget. In contrast, the government's Animal Damage Control Operations Program that financially supports the trapping and poisoning of coyotes and other livestock predators, received $26.6 million. A budget cut of $6.3 million for 1996 entails relying more on state and private entities to control damage to livestock by predators.

The Clinton administration proposed for fiscal year 1996 some $1.1 million for finalizing the necessary standards, accreditation rules, and implementation of the Organic Food Production Act. This act would establish national standards and certification of organic crop and animal produce. This is a result of public pressure and due to the fact that growth in the sales of organic produce have exceeded 20 percent for five consecutive years, and annual sales have topped $5 billion.

Government funding to encourage advances in the understanding and research assessment of farm animal well-being has been considerable in many European countries, especially in the United Kingdom and Germany. However, funding of such research is virtually *nonexistent* in the United States. Of the $8,476,952 awarded by the National Research Initiative (NRI) in 1994 through its "Sustaining Animal Health and Well-Being" program, $255,000 or a mere 3 percent went to research primarily concerned with animal well-being.

One of the lynchpins for information exchange and research data retrieval is the National Agricultural Library. Its Animal Welfare Information Center is an invaluable resource. At its inception the budget included $750,000 exclusively for the center's use. (For a comprehensive list of organizations and publications, see Resources at the end of this book.)

Chapter Four

Genetic Engineering and Biomedical Research

A cow is nothing but cells on the hoof.

Thomas Wagner, veterinary biotechnologist

G enetic engineering has become a scientific playground, and in the food industry it is a new technological fix for agriculture.[1] It entails inserting one or more genes from one life-form into another. For example, extra genes inserted into lambs, pigs, and fish make them grow faster; flounder fish antifreeze genes are placed into salmon so they can survive freezing waters; firefly genes are put into plants as genetic markers; genes from bacteria viruses and from certain plants are placed into corn, tomato, and squash so that these plants will be resistant to various diseases and herbicides; and genes from scorpions and spiders help make plants poisonous to insects. Genetic scientists also experiment with human genes, placing them in sheep, pigs, and cows for extensive experimentation to create new pharmaceuticals, or animal organs for human use.

Venture capitalists are investing heavily in biotechnology, which is rapidly changing the countryside and the animal kingdom as we know it. Genetic engineers are turning crops and farm animals into pharmaceutical factories and making natural foods a thing of the past. Scientists in private laboratories and corporate-funded universities are developing a whole new generation of life-forms. This new technology threatens to turn what is left of the countryside into what I call a bio-industrialized wasteland.

Genetically engineered foods are already available in the grocery store. However, consumers may not be able to identify them because the Food and Drug Administration (FDA) refuses to consider labeling for these types of food. In time, genetic engineering will radically change food ingredients and feedstuffs for the genetically engineered animals we will eat. These new animals will live in vast factories and provide us with meat, eggs, and dairy products, as well as pharmaceuticals, human blood, and organ parts. Already, engineered pigs can produce human blood. And because other genetically engineered pigs have immune systems similar to humans, they can serve as donors for people in need of a new heart, pancreas, or liver.

Agribusiness dismisses the fact that genetically engineered traits such as herbicide resistance, insect and virus resistance, stress tolerance and nitrogen-fixing ability can, and have, backfired. It is highly possible that the new traits might transfer from crops via their pollen to weeds through hybridization, and insects would quickly develop resistance. The end result would be even more troublesome weeds and insect pests.

Despite these risks, the USDA allows the release of genetically engineered crops and has virtually eliminated federal permits for field testing in order to speed bioengineered products to the market. All field testers need to do is notify the USDA of the intended field test. By December 1994, in spite of potential risks, the federal government under the flag of scientific field trials approved more than 2,250 deliberate test releases of genetically engineered organisms into the environment. I wonder what these new field trials will accomplish.

The Environmental Protection Agency (EPA) has the task of regulating the release of genetically engineered bacterial pesticides under the same rules developed to ensure the safe use of chemical pesticides. It is absurd to use the same rules, because chemical pesticides cannot reproduce and multiply like bacteria.

It is not farfetched to imagine a menu that includes a variety of genetically engineered products. These designer-food products will variously resist frost—such as tomatoes and strawberries containing fish antifreeze genes—and will have a longer shelf life. This means too that they will look fresh even if essential nutrients have long since deteriorated.

A Dinner of Transgenic Foods

Appetizers
Spiced Potatoes with Waxmoth gene
Juice of Tomatoes with Flounder gene

Entrée

Blackened Catfish with Trout gene
Scalloped Potatoes with Chicken gene
Cornbread with Firefly gene

Dessert

Rice Pudding with Pea gene

Beverage

Milk from Recombinant Bovine Growth Hormone (rBGH)-
supplemented Cows

(Federal permits for environmental release are pending or have been granted for all the transgenic plants and animals included on the menu. BGH is approved as a veterinary drug.)[2]

Sadly, I am unable to find any evidence that agricultural biotechnology is being used to *improve* the quality of the environment, or the well-being of farm animals. Nor is it being used to help alleviate world hunger. However, it is possible that the new generation of genetically engineered vaccines and disease diagnostic kits can help prevent animal and human illnesses and suffering.

No Protection for Farm Animals

Today, farm animals are being subjected to genetic engineering but the public know little about the widespread use of these animals in biomedical research. Animals used for genetic engineering or for biomedical research are not protected by the act. The Animal Welfare Act of the United States specifically excludes animals raised for food or fiber. With no real protection of farm animals at federal or state levels, abuse and cruelty of farm animals is widespread and legal.[3] Their welfare criteria seem to be dictated by current food and fiber production standards—which are abysmally inadequate for any animal—rather than by standards presently applicable to other warm-blooded animals in the Animal Welfare Act.

Farm animals have made valuable contributions as models in biomedical research, but have received little ethical consideration.[4] In Fiscal Year 1990, almost 67,000 farm animals were used in biomedical research; by Fiscal Year 1994, that number had jumped to nearly 180,667 with a notable 10 percent increase since 1993, according to the United States Department of Agriculture's Animal and Plant Health Inspection Service.

Poultry is probably the most popular of all farm animal models, being used for studies of arthritis, cardiovascular disease, viral infections like AIDS, and vaccine testing. Sheep are the second most frequently used farm animal in biomedical research. Beyond provision of a continuous resource for embryonic and fetal studies, experiments on sheep range from the testing of intrauterine devices and cardiac valves to viral disease observations, particularly that of the slow virus, scrapie, which is an excellent model for two human slow-virus infections, Creutzfeldt-Jakob disease and Kuru. Calves have almost entirely replaced dogs in heart transplantation studies, which dominate the field of tissue and organ transplantation started almost fifty years ago.

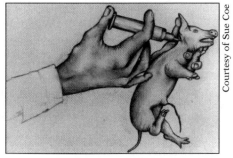

Courtesy of Sue Coe

Pigs are considered to be the farm animal model with greatest human similarity. Pediatricians and neonatologists love baby pigs' adherence to the anatomical growth curve of human newborns, and have used thousands of them to evaluate infant formulas and milk substitutes, diets for rehabilitation of infants with protein and calorie malnutrition, and the effect of severe malnutrition in early life on future learning abilities. Older pigs are used as models for gastric ulcers, skin-burn studies, wound healing, cardiovascular diseases, alcoholism, and tumor research.

The use of goats is on the rise in large part due to the ease with which they are handled, fed, and housed. The quality of antiserum and antitoxins produced by goats rivals that produced by rabbits; therefore, there is an economic advantage to using larger goat volumes. One of the more hideous uses of goats is their intentional wounding with bullets at Fort Bragg, North Carolina. This is an example of a poorly conceived animal experimentation intended to help train military medical surgeons. Once the anaesthetized goats are wounded they are operated on, and then euthanized before coming out of the anesthesia.

The pharmaceutical industry exploits horses as the number-one animal for hormone-replacement for menopausal women and osteoporosis prevention. The most notable product is Premarin manufactured by Wyeth-Ayerst Laboratories, which is taken by more than eight million women. About forty-two thousand horses are made pregnant annually. For six months of the eleven-month pregnancy, each mare is confined to a small stall, wearing a harness and a bag for urine collection. Some of the foals are raised for horse meat and exported live to

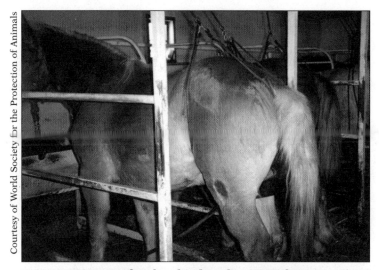

Courtesy of World Society for the Protection of Animals

Mare confined and tethered on PMU farm.

Japan for "fresh" slaughter. The life span of a mare can be from twenty to thirty years, but for a mare on a PMU (pregnancy mare urine) farm, their life span is decreased. Many can break down after nine or ten years on line. Additionally, they are subjected to lack of exercise, constant pregnancy, and injury.

For women looking for alternatives to Premarin, there are other products derived from plants instead of from mares. For example, the authors of *Natural Medicine for Menopause and Beyond*, suggest black cohosh. They note that black cohosh has been used in clinical practice for more than thirty-five years, especially in Germany. They report, "A randomized double-blind study proved that 4 mg. of black cohosh per day was superior to that of the usual daily dose of prescription conjugated estrogens such as Premarin in relieving menopausal symptoms."[5] (See Resources at the end of this book for the Women's International Pharmacy, a source for education and services for natural hormone replacement.)

Who Controls the Food? Who Knows What We Eat?

Beyond the serious concerns of creating designer foods, there is an even more disturbing issue that remains unseen: *Who* controls agriculture, and ultimately, what people can and cannot eat? *Who* controls the choices that consumers have in the marketplace? And what freedom do farmers have over what they grow and how they farm?

Other questions arise: Will these genetic changes pose a risk to consumers? Will they offend ethical and religious sensibilities? Would the antifreeze genes of fish—spliced into the genetic structure of strawberries and other fruits and vegetables to increase frost resistance—harm people who are allergic to fish? Will genetically engineered foods expose consumers to a host of new and unsuspected allergens? No one knows. Will these changes be an affront to Jains, Hindus, and other ethical vegetarians?

Yet another concern arises over *what* plant and animal varieties farmers can raise. The monopolistic control by corporations has the potential of shifting the decision-making process from the farmers, who know the land best, to the corporate boardrooms of food industry conglomerates. The outcome of their decisions is likely to be fueled primarily by greed, considering the direction being taken by agribusiness as it multiplies and diversifies its investments in biotechnology.

It is essential that food industry *label all genetically engineered foods*. Labeling gives consumers information to *choose* in the marketplace. Labels will enable consumers to refuse to buy foods that they believe are suspect and to support those farmers, food retailers, and processors who value natural foods and sustainable farming.

It is a well-known fact that pesticides injure consumer health and the environment. However, agribusiness corporations that are now investing in agricultural biotechnology have long denied, and even covered up, the harmful consequences of pesticides. This is one reason why agribusiness forcefully lobbies against the labeling of genetically engineered foods and food additives. If genetically engineered foods prove to be dangerous, they do not want to be held responsible.

Agribusiness corporations are not going to have farmers change the way they raise crops and livestock in order to reduce pesticide and animal drug dependence until they have a market for their next generation of costly alternative products, especially the patented products of genetic engineering biotechnology. Agribusiness corporations have put their own vested interest in selling pesticides before considering the public interest in safe and wholesome food. How can we trust agribusiness corporations to protect the public interest when it comes to genetically engineered foods? Furthermore, how can we expect state and federal agencies to effectively regulate agricultural biotechnology when such agencies have failed abysmally to effectively regulate pesticide and antibiotic use?

The media have given spotty and incomplete coverage to a public interest and policy issue that entails a *fundamental* change in the nature of the food we eat. Genes pass from one generation to the next. Change the genetic composition of tomatoes, apples, and pigs, then all the tomatoes, apples, and pork that we eat in the years and generations to come could be different. The media have superficially glossed over these consumer-related concerns about genetically altered foods, dubbing them "Frankenfoods." The media report in detail on the widely hyped biotechnology industry's promises of safer, more nutritious, even more palatable fruits, vegetables, and animal products that will spoil slowly, if at all. But who will ask the tough questions and get to the roots of consumers' concerns?

Concerns and Doubts About Biotechnology

Consumers are quite concerned about the socio-economic impacts of biotechnology on farmers and rural communities. A 1992 interim report by the USDA's Extension Service revealed some significant public perceptions and attitudes.[6] The survey found that:

♦ 85 percent of those surveyed feel it is important to label foods if biotechnology is used;

♦ 94 percent want to know if pesticides are used;

♦ 88 percent want labels on irradiated foods;

♦ 24 percent feel that the use of biotechnology to alter plants is morally wrong;

♦ 53 percent feel it is morally wrong to alter animals, and expressed more concern over eating meat and dairy products developed with biotechnology than eating genetically engineered fruits and vegetables;

♦ Consumer acceptance of plant-to-plant genetic engineering is 66 percent; however, it fell drastically to 39 percent acceptance of genetic engineering for animal-to-animal, and only 10 per cent approval for human-to-animal transgenic alteration.

Biotechnology proponents point out that genetic engineering holds enormous promise for the cure of human diseases, fostering human life, and reducing suffering. While the medical benefits of appropriate biotechnology are considerable, there are three major concerns to address.

♦ Are companies using technology to bioengineer humankind to live in an increasingly polluted environment, just as is being done to farm animals?

♦ What about the suffering of animals genetically engineered to serve as models for human diseases?

♦ What does bioengineering contribute to the overall quality of life for the human species?

Proponents claim biotechnology could play a beneficial role in sustainable agriculture. But this claim needs to be examined. There are three basic approaches to enhance animal health and productivity using this new technology that we need to question. They are gene splicing, embryonic transfer, and cloning.

Gene Splicing

Gene-spliced bacteria have the ability to manufacture new-generation animal vaccines and pharmaceuticals. Examples are interferon, which boosts immunity, and growth hormones, which boost growth rates and milk yield. Manufacturers claim growth hormones are analogs of natural compounds already present in the animal's body. Various plants, including tobacco, bananas, and tomatoes, for example, have been gene-spliced to produce similar pharmaceutical products and even vaccines for future medical and veterinary application. The safety and efficacy of products of biotech "pharming" is still an unknown. They are analogous (as distinct from homologous) products.

In other words, analogs are not entirely natural. We need to question their use in farm animals to artificially enhance immunity, disease resistance, growth rate, muscle-mass, and milk yield.

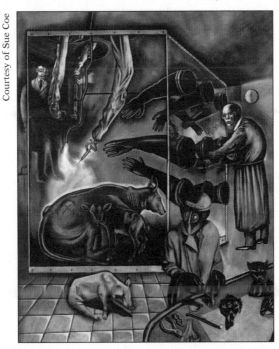

Courtesy of Sue Coe

Manufacturers are currently developing and marketing gene-spliced bacteria for feeding to pigs and for injection into the rumens or first stomachs of cattle. These bacteria are supposed to help improve the digestibility of various nonfood feed ingredients, such as sawdust and newspaper pulp. Aside from the health issues for the animals ingesting sawdust and newspaper pulp, the animal and consumer health risks are considerable. These new bacteria also pose potentially harmful environmental effects when the bacteria are excreted in animal manure.

Gene-spliced, so-called "transgenic farm animals," are being developed, but their commercial future is at least five years to ten years away. Transgenic farm animals are being created to be primarily more productive rather than disease- or stress-resistant or to produce pharmaccutical products in their milk. Biotechnologists are creating transgenic farm animals and fish by inserting the genes of other species, including human genes, or extra genes of the animals' own kind, into their developing embryos. Some of the transgenic animals will be able to transmit these additional genes to their offspring.

What will be the implications of additional genes entering the gene pool of a species? How do biotechnologists control this? These questions have not been answered. The technology bounding forward without first carefully considering the inherent problems and finding solutions is reminiscent of the nuclear energy industry.

Many biomedical research industry laboratories are using this technology to create transgenic animals afflicted with defective human genes. Biogeneticists will then develop birth defects, cancer, brain tumors, and other diseases that will cause the animals much suffering. This will lead to testing new drugs on the animals for the inflicted disease. This is ethically and scientifically questionable in terms of "real progress" in human medicine. And *who* will oversee and regulate the extent of experimenting done on animals in this new scientific playground?

Embryo Transfer and Cloning

Biotechnology looks to developments in embryo transfer and cloning as the answers to increased animal production and health. However, these developments potentially can create a loss of genetic diversity in the farm animal population. The result is the selection of varieties of livestock and poultry suited only to intensive production systems. In terms of overall animal health and well-being, biotechnology products are developed primarily for intensive, factory farming production systems. Long-term social and economic consequences on the structure and future of agriculture are therefore considerable.

In March 1997, the news media around the world splashed the story of the British scientist, Ian Wilmut, who successfully engineered the first clone of a mammal, a sheep, from an adult cell. Wilmut used a cell taken from the udder tissue of a sheep, fused it into an egg and implanted it into the womb of a surrogate ewe. This sheep's replica, named "Dolly," was born.

As of mid-1997, only twenty-nine of some 277 sheep embryos cloned by Wilmut developed normally. Many died before birth, had defective kidneys, or were abnormally large—not the exact replicas the biotechnologist had anticipated. Such high death and disability rates in creating transgenic animals have not been regulated, nor seriously addressed in most research reports.

This new technology brings us to the threshold of human cloning and a myriad of ethical questions and fears. Most important, what is the point in cloning animals? And second, where might it all lead? The technique developed by Wilmut has been patented, and venture capitalists have high hopes that cloning will be a boost to the organ transplant industry and to pharmaceutical "pharming" of health care products. Pigs, sheep, cattle, and goats have already been genetically engineered to serve as organ donors for people. They can also produce more humanlike milk and milk containing valuable biopharmaceuticals. The numbers of these animals used might now be rapidly increased using cloning technology.

One serious problem with creating animal clones is that, because of their genetic conformity, they are more likely to be vulnerable to infectious diseases. Another problem is the suffering of animals afflicted by genetic and developmental defects caused *accidentally*—because the technology is not risk-free—or else the defects were *deliberately* caused in order to research genetic and developmental diseases. Already hundreds of varieties of genetically engineered mice have been created, many with such defects. Under the present federal Animal Welfare Act rodents are excluded from any protection, therefore their suffering is not taken into consideration.

Courtesy of Sue Coe

Another ethical issue of cloning is that the ever-intensifying commercial exploitation of animals will lead to regarding these living beings as "biomachines." Many fear that animals will become primarily a source of replacement body fluids and parts for humans—from blood and bones to livers and hearts. These valuable patented human creations—"manimals"—of the new industrial biofarms of the next century could serve a wealthy elite. "Manimals" could provide replacement body parts and vital elements as needed.

Cloning advocates may claim this biotechnology could help save endangered species by facilitating their replication in captivity. But can we preserve the natural by such unnatural means? And all to what end?

Cloning transgenic animals to manufacture new biopharmaceuticals preempts the development of humane production technologies. Commercial-scale cloning will reinforce the demeaning perception of animals as disposable commodities of human creation. Patenting cloned, genetically engineered animals further erodes the ethic of respect for the intrinsic value and sanctity of individual life, an ethical principle that is critical to the future well-being of both humans and other animals.

Animals must be on the agenda of human concern. Until they are, cloning and other developments in biotechnology are likely to do more harm than good and serve the interests of an increasingly depraved corporate agenda. The bioethical questions about how far we can and should go in interfering with nature, with life, and with the earth's creation, have yet to be openly and fairly addressed. For now, humans need to have more compassion for animals rather than taking the next step—cloning—which is another inhumane act toward animals.

Who Needs Recombinant Bovine Growth Hormone?

Genetically engineered bovine growth hormone (rBGH) is the first product that the biotechnology industry has yet to recognize as their Ford Edsel. It is not necessary or beneficial. Yet, the FDA has bent over backwards to get rBGH (recombinant bovine growth hormone) approved for injection into dairy cows to boost milk production. Despite unresolved consumer health and animal welfare concerns and chronic oversupplies of milk, the FDA has pushed for the use of rBGH. *Why?*

In 1993 I testified before an FDA panel in Rockville, Maryland during a series of regional public hearings on rBGH. Its task was to weigh the pros and cons of injecting dairy cows with rBGH. (Another name for this product is recombinant bovine somatotropin [rBST].) The manufacturers of rBGH attested to its safety to cows and consumers. They repeatedly touted the efficacy and cost savings of rBGH under good management. My testimony was as follows:

> I wish to go on record as being opposed to FDA approval of genetically engineered recombinant bovine growth hormone (rBGH) until there is a valid assessment and resolution to the mastitis (infection of the cow's udder) issue. I have reviewed published reports on the effects of rBGH on commercial dairy cows. These reports show a clear correlation between husbandry factors that contribute to dairy cow diseases and the use of rBGH. These diseases, especially mastitis, will be predictably exacerbated by rBGH treatment.

The drug, rBGH, essentially hyperstimulates the dairy cow to produce more milk, which can lower the animal's disease resistance and contribute to increased incidence of lameness and mastitis. Profound physiological changes can also lead to metabolic disorders and reproductive problems, notably infertility. We think that the incorporation of rBGH into dairy cow husbandry is likely to create an opportunistic niche for viral and mycoplasma disease. This could become a costly endemic problem in the nation's dairy herd, especially in view of the potential immunosuppressive effects of rBGH.

Alternative husbandry practices, such as rotational grazing, will increase productivity without jeopardizing dairy cow health and welfare. If FDA approves rBGH, we will consider supporting a nationwide boycott of all dairy products until FDA mandates labeling of products derived from cows not injected with this hormone. There are also adverse socio-economic consequences to small- and midsize dairy farmers. We cannot overlook public health concerns (especially over the unresolved question of insulin-like growth factor in rBGH milk). There are consumer-right-to-know issues arising from the specter of rBGH being injected into the nation's dairy herd.

We should not overlook the most obvious economic inefficiency of using rBGH to increase milk production. When farmers use rBGH they have to feed their cows more costly high-energy concentrate feeds. This wastes the natural ability of the dairy cow to efficiently convert low nutrient plant material into milk protein for human consumption. The incorporation of any genetically engineered product like rBGH into the food production system is a backward step indeed.

Finally, the public equates milk with purity. Public support will erode if the dairy industry adopts the use of rBGH. The public is well aware that antibiotic milk-residues will become more of a problem because of an increase in mastitis in the national herd paralleling increasing use of rBGH.

Clearly, rBGH is a product that is beyond the FDA's scope of objective, science-based evaluation. Its approval rests upon a regulatory framework that in theory purports to protect consumer health and safety, but in practice would be so costly to effectively enforce. Costly enforcement at public expense would negate any purported savings to the public of a cheap and plentiful supply of milk from rBGH-treated cows.

Quite simply, rBGH is a bad choice and a poor start for the biotechnocrats. Seemingly without thinking, and against overwhelming evidence to the contrary, the FDA went ahead and approved rBGH as safe. The FDA further accommodated the manufacturers by ruling that milk and dairy products from treated cows does not merit or need labeling.

As predicted, a number of dairy farmers who have used rBGH to increase their herd's milk production now regret the move. John Shumway of western New York said his herd started to develop severe mastitis problems shortly after he started the rBGH shots. He has had to sell a quarter of his cows. "It has been devastating," he reported. Charles Knight, a Florida farmer, experienced an immediate production boost upon giving the shots. Then his herd's health declined. After two months of rBGH shots, the cooperative wouldn't accept his farm's milk because of its high pus content. He finally stopped using rBGH after losing nine cows.

Sources at the Wisconsin Farmers Union say they have received reports from farmers in seven different states who experienced herd health problems after using the drug.[7] "Over the last six months, adverse reaction reports filed with the FDA have jumped over 800 percent," according to Mark A. Kastel, director of Governmental Affairs with the Wisconsin Farmers Union.[8] In the majority of these cases, reports reflect problems "with many cows and multiple disorders on a given farm." Problems reported to both the FDA and the Wisconsin Farmers Union hotline have included the death of cows, incurable mastitis, hoof and leg maladies, infections, breeding problems, and internal bleeding.

Kastel says that one farmer who milks approximately two hundred cows in Lisbon, New York, is one of many farmers who has related "horror stories" to the Farmers Union. "For the first couple of months on rBST our cows seemed to be doing okay. Their milk production increased from forty to sixty-five pounds per day...then they just went all to pieces!" exclaimed farmer Jay Livingston. "We had a half-dozen cows die, and then the rest started experiencing major health problems. Cows went off their feed, experienced severe weight loss, mastitis, and serious foot problems."

Jay Livingston continued by saying, "Initially, we went to a meeting co-sponsored by Monsanto and our veterinarian. They came and checked out our herd and said everything was rosy, that this rBST is the greatest thing since sliced bread. We did just what they told us to do.

"When we started to develop problems, a representative from the corporation that produces rBST, a representative from Monsanto came out to the farm and told us we were the only ones having problems. They blamed us and had every excuse from here to hell and back, but totally rejected that rBST had any relationship to our problems." Livingston, who farms with his brother, stated that his family has never had herd health problems before taking the vet's recommendation and going on rBST.

After losing more than $100,000 in milk sales—and having to replace fifty cows that either died or had to be put down—Kastel said, "Mr. Livingston is understandably bitter. He always had quality milk with a somatic cell count of one hundred thousand to one hundred fifty thousand. When we were on rBST, it went up to seven hundred thousand or more. They should outlaw this stuff!"

Even though the Livingston farm has not used rBST since June 1994, many of the treated cows are now having problems while giving birth. During a two-month period of time, the Livingstons had twenty cows give birth to twins, which is abnormal. Virtually none of the calves survived, and the mortality rate of the mothers is approximately 50 percent. "This is just one of over eight hundred horror stories that are now on record," Kastel reported.

Kastel said Monsanto has also engaged in a practice of issuing $150 vouchers for veterinary care to farmers who initially ordered rBGH. "One hundred fifty dollars may seem rather innocuous until you realize that some of these veterinary practices have pushed rBGH very hard and have fifty to one hundred dairy farms signed up. Now we're talking about many thousands of dollars, and we relate to this as a blatant kickback to the veterinarians."

Bruce Krug is a Constableville, New York, farmer and coordinator of the New York Farmers Union. He is researching the fact that New York, among many other states, has statutes that prohibit veterinarians from taking any "direct or indirect" compensation from pharmaceutical companies to promote their products. According to Krug, Monsanto has underwritten joint promotional campaigns with veterinary clinics in an effort to sell farmers on rBGH. The Farmers Union is presently trying to verify whether or not these promotion efforts and this financial compensation constitute a violation of law.

Interestingly, not only are veterinarians being compensated through Monsanto's voucher program, but according to farmer Livingston, they are also profiting from their customers' rBGH usage. "After our problems started in April and May, we experienced over a three thousand dollar vet bill! "explained Livingston. "After discontinuing rBGH usage, our vet bill went to virtually zero. We didn't even see the vet for six weeks."

Consumers' Right to Know Versus FDA Agenda

According to recent polls, 80 percent of United States consumers show concern about the human health hazards of foods from cows injected with rBGH, and more than 90 percent of dairy farmers have refused to use the drug. Consumer and farmer support for rBGH-free products is evident not only in the United States, but also in the European Community and Canada. The European Union, which includes fifteen countries, has extended its moratorium on the commercial use of rBGH through the year 1999.

The FDA has ignored reports that rBGH treatment can make cows sick and infertile, and that antibiotic residues to treat these sick cows passes on through their milk and puts consumers at risk. The FDA insists that it has established an adequate regulatory structure to ensure consumer safety of all genetically engineered fruits, vegetables, and animal products. Therefore, the FDA feels labeling these new foods will serve no useful purpose.

In poll after poll, 70 percent to 90 percent of United States consumers indicate that they *want* labels on the milk that comes from rBGH-injected cows. Yet the public's right to choose rBGH-free dairy products has not prevailed because the FDA refuses to mandate the labeling of all products from treated cows. Clearly, the FDA—which is ostensibly responsible for protecting the public—has sided with the manufacturers and is ignoring the public. In opposition to the FDA's decision, fourteen states currently have legislative bills introduced for labeling rBGH milk and dairy products even though they risk massive lawsuits from Monsanto, the rBGH manufacturer.

The human health risks of increased levels of insulin-like growth factor in the milk of cows treated with rBGH are considerable. In an extensive review of many scientific studies, physician Samuel Epstein concludes that the milk of these cows is likely to cause, or increase susceptibility to breast and colon cancer in humans. Developing human fetuses, children, and adolescents, may be especially at risk.[9]

The rationale for denying consumers' right to know that dairy products have come from rBGH-treated cows was developed by then-Deputy FDA Commissioner Michael Taylor in 1993. Before joining the FDA, he was a former chief counsel for the International Food Biotechnology Council and the agribusiness corporation, Monsanto. Anticipated profits for Monsanto from rBGH were never realized, since by 1996 only 10 percent of the nation's dairy herd was being injected. In spite of Monsanto's claims to the contrary, more and more dairy farmers who had used rBGH were no longer using it.

Genetic Engineering Versus Organic Agriculture

Conventional breeding techniques in farm animals is far better than gene splicing. We can refine conventional breeding techniques by genetic screening and by using the untapped genetic resources of rare and minor breeds of livestock and poultry. The American Livestock Breeds Conservancy of Pittsboro, North Carolina, has worked for many years to preserve as many of the old breeds of livestock and poultry as possible. This preserved animal gene pool will be of extreme importance in livestock and poultry breeding as we re-establish more sustainable, ecological farming systems, where farm animals are better adapted to local conditions and free ranging rather than confined in factories and feedlots.

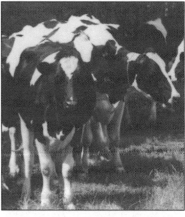

Photo: Michael W. Fox

There are, of course, limitations in traditional breeding practices that rely on the relatively narrow genetic base of most commercial varieties of livestock and poultry. There is some question if it is acceptable to employ biotechnology to enhance adaptability, including disease resistance and higher digestibility in animals developed for organic farming and ranching systems. For example, genetic resistance to *coccidiosis*, an intestinal parasite in poultry, may be forthcoming from some rare variety or wild member of the same species. Gene mapping, improved selective breeding, and embryo transfer biotechnologies hold greater promise to improve disease resistance and adaptability to future organic farming systems than bioengineering. Genetic engineering of crop varieties and farm animals has no place in organic agriculture, and any product labeled "organic" should certainly not have been subjected to biogenetic engineering.

Biotechnologists reason that one of the criteria for organic farming is the use of natural products. This includes using natural rather than synthetic chemical fertilizers. Biotechnologists feel, then, that transgenic crop varieties should be eligible for organic certification since the foreign genes they contain from other life-forms are "natural" in origin. This same line of reasoning would accept genetically engineered recombinant DNA products such as biopesticides and bovine and porcine growth hormones as natural and thus acceptable under organic farming and food standards. This reasoning is flawed since such bioengineered products and processes do not naturally occur or exist in conventional crops and animals.

Genetically engineered microorganisms for waste treatment (bioremediation) or to improve digestive efficiency, especially of cellulose and phosphate, should not be used because their short- and long-term risks are *unknown*. Further, we should not use these microorganisms to reduce waste emission problems such as ruminant methane and fecal nitrates in livestock and poultry. These kinds of high-cost inputs and correctives are not naturally intrinsic, ecologically compatible, or in accord with the philosophy and science of organic agriculture.

Bioethical Criteria

All developments in biotechnology need rigorous evaluation. I developed the following bioethical criteria to evaluate the new technology. Creating an International Bioethics Council within the United Nations would be a beginning to help ensure that this new technology be applied with the minimum of harm.

♦ **Necessity. Is the new technology, product or service really necessary, safe and effective? Are there alternatives of lesser risk and cost?**

♦ Public demand and acceptance.

♦ Environmental impact, short- and long-term, and influence on wild plant and animal (including invertebrate) species and microorganisms.

♦ Can released genetically engineered life forms be identified, traced, contained, or recalled if needed?

♦ Economic impact, social justice, and equity (international and intergenerational). Who will benefit? Who might be harmed?

♦ Animal welfare. Will the new product or service enhance farm animal health and overall well-being?

♦ Social and cultural consequences, such as impact on the structure of agriculture, nationally and internationally, and on more sustainable, traditional and alternative agricultural practices at home and abroad.

♦ Oversight and compliance. Can the new technology, product or service be effectively regulated to maximize benefits and minimize risks, and at what cost to society?

Big business agriculture is not sustainable, and agri-biotechnology is being misapplied as a profitable remedy for fundamentally unsound farming practices. I believe we need to change these unsound practices, *not* the genetic structure of crops and farm animals.

Chapter Five

A Sea of Troubled Waters:

Factory Fishing and Aquaculture

*The glory of the human has become the
desolation of the earth. This I would consider an
appropriate way to summarize the twentieth century.*

Thomas Berry, theologian

M any people are turning to fish and other seafood as an alternative
to meat and poultry. Fish consumption is rising. According to the
U.S. Department of Agriculture, Americans are eating more fish, estimated in 1993 at fifteen pounds per person, and spending $38 billion
on seafood per year. However, there are some serious health, environmental, and humane concerns to consider. Until recently, seafood was
not subject to inspection regulations by the United States government.

It is not an overstatement to say that marine fisheries are the world's
fastest dwindling resource. Overfishing, along with ocean pollution,
threaten to eliminate the United States coastal fin-fish stocks. According
to the United Nation's Food and Agriculture Organization (FAO), "Global
fish production from most marine resources and many inland waters has
reached or exceeded the level of maximum sustainable yield."

Overfishing

Overfishing by factory boats is turning the oceans into aquatic
deserts. Advanced fishing methods that include sonar, driftnets, and
floating refrigerated fish packing factories are pushing one species
after another to the edge of extinction. Inadequate international
enforcement of fishing quotas is decimating the world fish population.

In one of the first major newspaper articles on this subject, published in 1994, *Washington Post* reporter Anne Swardson addressed the critical status of the world's fishery resources:

♦ About 60 percent of the fish types tracked by the Food and Agriculture Organization of the United Nations (FAO) are categorized as fully exploited, over-exploited, or depleted.

♦ Meanwhile, the world population—the people who would eat these fish—is growing. On a per capita basis, the global catch of fish from all sources fell from 42.8 pounds in 1988 to 39.7 pounds in 1992. One reason predominates: over-fishing.[1]

Some of the first people to be hurt by overfishing are the world's poor, especially coastal peoples in developing countries. These people often rely on fish as their primary source of protein. Fish supplies 6.6 percent of the animal protein consumed in North America, 12 percent in Europe, 19 percent in Africa, and 29 percent in Asia. As fish stocks decline worldwide, those people most dependent upon seafood will be the first to suffer.

The FAO calculates that commercial fishers spend $120 billion worldwide each year to catch $70 billion worth of fish. Government subsidies make up most of the difference, thus encouraging overfishing. The fifteen-nation European Union spends some $580 million in annual fishing subsidies. Norway alone subsidizes its fishers with $150 million annually. Reportedly the Japanese have extended $19 billion in credit to its fishing industry, much of which the Japanese fishers will never pay back.

The recent closing of six thousand square miles of George's Bank fishing grounds off New England because of overfishing, and the Clinton administration's grant of $50 million to the New England fishing industry, are drastic steps predicated by decades of irresponsible mismanagement of wild fish stocks by the fishing industry. Using public funds to help fishers make ends meet when they have helped put themselves out of business by not regulating how much fish they catch seems wrong. The government needs to play a proactive role to protect fishing grounds from overfishing and from the harms of agrichemical runoff and municipal industrial pollution.

Many people are aware of the cruel killing of dolphins by yellowfin tuna fishers and purchase tuna with the *Dolphin Safe* label. Trade embargoes imposed in 1990 were due to the outcry over the tuna fishers' use of huge encircling purse-seine nets that killed hundreds of thousands of dolphins a year. However, the *Dolphin Safe* label is no longer worth looking for since the Clinton administration in 1997 gave the go-ahead for Mexico and ten other countries (Belize, Colombia, Costa Rica, Ecuador, France, Honduras, Panama, Spain, Vanuatu, and Venezuela) to import tuna to the United States that use fishing methods that are *not* dolphin safe.

Until the United Nations moratorium on driftnets of 1992, high seas nations with government-approved driftnet fleets included China, Taiwan, South Korea, Japan (on a smaller scale: France, Italy, and the United Kingdom). These countries had gigantic fishing fleet factories that used miles and miles of driftnets to virtually empty the oceans of life. According to DriftNetwork of Earthtrust, during the 1989 driftnet season over fifty whales were taken by the Taiwanese in the Indian Ocean. There are no patrols in this ocean, which is a sperm whale sanctuary. Although there is a moratorium on this type of fishing, illegal fishing continues with little concern by governments to enforce the ban.

According to the United States National Oceanic and Atmospheric Administration, in 1990 driftnetters ensnared approximately forty-two million marine mammals, seabirds and other non-target species while harvesting squid and tuna. Shrimp trawlers may have a higher rate of by-catch, pulling in from 80 percent to 90 percent "trash" fish with each haul. In most cases, they dump the trash fish back into the sea, many injured and/or dying.

Much of the catch from the sea goes to meet the increasing demand for feed on fish farms. Factory boats often harvest krill and "coarse" (poor quality eating) fish to use as feed for livestock, poultry, and fish farms. Krill is a vital food source for some marine mammals, including whales. Some 60 percent to 70 percent of the world's fish catch goes to livestock as a high-protein fish meal supplement, or for use as fertilizer. Fish meal comes from fish considered unsuitable for human consumption and the remains of fish processed for the fish market. This is a high-protein feed supplement for livestock, poultry, farmed fish, and pet food.

Unfortunately, since fish are in a highly contaminated environment, so is their food chain. Their bodies become loaded with pollutants. Predictably, mercury in the fish of some commercial cat food has caused measurable neurological and behavioral changes in felines. Marine mammals such as polar bears, walruses, whales, dolphins, and seals concentrate many chemical pollutants in their bodies because they consume vast quantities of various seafood. This may, in part, account for their declining fertility, weakened immune systems, and disease epidemics. In the spring of 1995 two whales beached and died on the coast of Belgium. Tests showed serious contamination in their bodies. The whale bodies fell under the legal definition of "toxic waste," which mandated their immediate incineration.

Reduced fish populations have had an impact on other marine life, most notable those that compete with humans for the fish. The fur seal industry uses the fact of dwindling fish catches to justify killing more seals. They blame the seals for contributing to the decline in fish stocks. Salmon farmers routinely kill hungry seals as they try to break into the floating salmon enclosures. Colonies of pelagic and coastal birds that include pelicans, petrels, puffins, and penguins are dwindling. These birds suffer from starvation, disease, and reproductive failure due to overfishing and pollution of the marine environment.

In addition to overfishing, soil erosion from deforested and agricultural land, along with the runoff of chemical fertilizers and pesticides, is contributing to the destruction of coastal waters and coral reefs, as well as inland lakes, rivers, and wetlands. A vast stretch of the Gulf of Mexico will not support life because of a condition called "hypoxia," meaning insufficient oxygen in body tissue. Fertilizers from the Mississippi Delta cause the ocean plankton to bloom, a phenomenon called "eutrophication". The plankton eventually die and sink to the bottom of the Gulf of Mexico where they decay. But because of their extremely high density, the decaying process consumes all the oxygen in the deep water. This wipes out bottom feeders such as shrimp and harms the entire ecology and economy of the gulf.

This continued abuse of the oceans will result in the oceans becoming a nonviable food source. It will be an even greater calamity if the nations of the world do nothing but focus on developing aquaculture as an alternative, rather than cooperating to restore marine ecosystems.

Journalist Anne Swardson writes, "Meanwhile millions of boats keep catching billions of fish. The march toward empty oceans leads Gus Newton of the FAO to joke that perhaps we should declare the high seas a kind of nature preserve. He half-envisions a watery international park in which we would ban fishing entirely. 'At least,' he said, sounding half-serious, 'then we'd have something left to show our children.'"[2]

Aquaculture, Aquabusiness: A Pharmaceutical Stew

Aquaculture or fish farming is a growing industry in the United States. Commercial fish farming will soon become the primary source of seafood to compensate for declining stocks of wild ocean fish. The intensive factory farming of seafood species and freshwater fish like trout, tilapia, and catfish increased from six and one half million tons in 1984 to thirteen million tons in 1991. This represents 13 percent of the total world consumption of seafood. In 1992 growers worldwide raised 720,000 tons of shrimp .

However, fish farming is actually hastening fish extinction by disrupting coastal ecosystems and by causing drug and chemical pollution from products used by commercial seafood producers.[3] In addition, fresh water fish, like those in the Great Lakes, are heavily contaminated with pesticides, heavy metals, PCBs, and dioxins. As a consequence, some species have failed to reproduce and are now extinct. Certain subspecies of the Pacific salmon are now facing extinction and much of the salmon consumed today comes from salmon farms in coastal waters of the Atlantic Ocean and North Sea

Further, intensive factory farming of salmon and other aquatic species causes a tremendous risk to aquatic life because of the antibiotics and other drugs that are fed to the farmed fish to control diseases. These chemicals remain in uneaten feed and fish excrement. A twenty-acre salmon farm produces as much waste as a town of ten thousand people. The American Society for Microbiology has recently targeted antibiotics used in aquaculture as a major global concern because it contributes to the spread of antibiotic-resistant bacteria in the ocean.

Growers use drugs, like the pesticide Dichlorovos to control disease such as sea lice. They often just pour the drugs over the salmon. Not only is it bad for the salmon but it could be harmful to all manner of ocean life.[4] These drugs, along with some of the diseases of aquaculture stock, threaten indigenous aquatic wildlife and their environment. Some fish species are migratory, thus posing the risk of carrying disease great distances after becoming infected from fish farm effluent. For example, in 1989 the wild sea trout fisheries off the west coast of Ireland collapsed. The sea trout suffered from sea lice and possibly other diseases contracted from infected salmon being raised nearby in overcrowded floating cages. The decline of herring in the Bay of Fundy coincides with the harmful ecological consequences of floating salmon fish farms.

According to aquaculture scientist Dr. F.P. Myers, disease problems constitute the largest single cause of economic losses in aquaculture. In 1988 channel catfish producers lost more than one hundred million fish, worth nearly $11 million. The trout industry reported 1988 losses of over twenty million fish worth over $2.5 million. He concludes that we "urgently need research to support the registration of promising therapeutic agents."[5] In other words, we need better surveillance of potentially harmful drugs that are now being widely used in aquaculture.

Aquaculture needs more effective food safety inspection because of the incredible number of different chemicals and drugs used to make cultured fish and shrimp productive. Fish farming is essentially raising creatures in a pharmaceutical stew.[6] A few of the chemicals used in aquaculture include: benzalkonium chloride, benzocaine, chloramine T, erythromycin, copper sulfate, formalin, hydrogen peroxide, oxytetracycline, potassium permanganate, and sarafloxacin; hormones such as human chorionic gonadotropin, methyl testosterone, luteinizing hormone releasing analogs, and carp pituitary extract. The FDA considers the following fish farming drugs high regulatory priority: certain bactericide-antibiotics; central nervous system stimulants and depressants; chloramphenicol; fluoroquinolones; nitrofurans; quinolones; certain steroid hormones. *Appetizing* isn't it?

Fish and shrimp farms in the developing world are causing grave ecological damage, especially destruction of mangrove swamps and pollution of coastal waters. These farms also require high energy protein feeds. This means less arable land is available to raise food for the people in developing countries, and few benefit financially from export-oriented aquaculture development programs.

However, compared to intensive livestock and poultry production, fish farming is more efficient and thus more appealing to investors and food producers. Consider the feed requirements for fish versus meat:

+ Growing a kilogram of beef typically takes seven kilograms of feed.

+ One kilogram of pork takes four kilograms of feed.

+ Even though chicken is the most efficient of all the land-based meats, it still takes two to two and one-half kilograms of feed for each kilogram of weight gain.

+ Fish is the most efficient. It takes one and one-half to two and one-half kilograms of feed, to raise one kilogram of fish.[7]

The aquaculture industry is now genetically engineering fish to grow faster.[8] These may be the first animal food products of biotechnology to reach the marketplace. However, genetically engineered fish may be more susceptible to stress, disease, and ultraviolet radiation, thus requiring more drugs to maintain health and productivity in aquaculture tanks and floating cages.

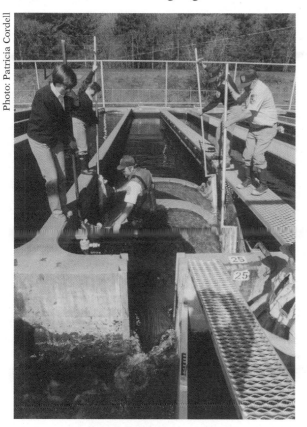

A fish hatchery in Oregon

Photo: Patricia Cordell

Fish Hatcheries

Fish hatcheries, primarily for trout and salmon production and release into streams and rivers for anglers, are a factory farming enterprise that *Washington Post* reporter Tom Kenworth describes as being "caught between the wisdom and politics of stocking."[9] Kenworth documents that many researchers have found that excessive reliance on hatcheries has led to the spread of disease to wild fish and a loss of genetic diversity.

Hatchery-raised stock may initially outcompete their wild cousins, killing them off through competition for food, and then die out because of their poorer resistance to stress and disease. The end result is less fish in our rivers. But anglers want their fish, and political pressure on hatcheries subsidized by anglers' licenses to maintain the status quo is considerable. Private sector and state hatchery reform is urgently needed, coupled with better protection and restoration of our waterways, wild fish populations, and other aquatic life.

Is Seafood Safe to Eat?

Consuming more fish and other seafood as an alternative protein source is a questionable choice in the United States and in other relatively affluent industrial countries. It is no exaggeration to see the oceans, especially coastal waters, as open sewers. Considering seafood as an alternate source of protein, may not be a wise choice. Fish easily absorb toxic chemicals. Many species of fish have unacceptable levels of various pesticides, dioxins, PCBs, cadmium, and mercury. It is well documented that PCBs and dioxins are considered a major cause of a host of human health problems from cancer and infertility to neurological problems such as attention deficit disorders and lower IQ in children.[10]

Until very recently, seafood has not been subject to any effective standards of food safety inspection and compliance in the United States. Fortunately, the Food and Drug Administration now mandates a HACCUP seafood inspection system. The FDA is required to inspect each of the country's six thousand fish processing plants at least once every three years and at most once a year. At inspection, samples are taken to be evaluated later. However, no regulations pertain to the one hundred thousand fishing vessels that haul in fish in the open seas and bring it to market.[11]

If you are going to eat fish, probably the safest seafood to consume are those in the middle of the food chain. The bottom feeders, such as the scavenging shrimp and crabs, and filter-feeding mollusks such as clams and oysters, concentrate various pollutants in their tissues. Commonly these are heavy metals such as lead, cadmium, mercury, PCBs, dioxins, and pesticides. Fish in the middle of the food chain such as herring and snapper generally ingest less harmful chemicals than the big fish at the top of the food chain, such as tuna and swordfish. Low-fat species such as cod, pollack, and haddock from far offshore, are safer, as are younger, smaller fish that have not lived long enough to accumulate contaminants.

Farmed fish, especially salmon, trout, catfish, and tilapia, along with crayfish, shrimps, and oysters, may seem like a safe alternative. These aquaculture products could promise a safe, less-contaminated food source provided growers produce them using few drugs and, ideally, organically. The problem of overfishing in the ocean would be alleviated only if fish farming is ecological.

As an alternative to fish, there is an abundance of highly nutritious proteins of vegetable origin, and eggs and dairy products from humanely raised animals. The health benefits a person hopes to achieve from eating fish as a source of omega-3 fatty acids can better be had from organic flax-seed oil and oil of primrose.

The health and welfare of intensively raised fish, as well as consumer risks of drug residues in the fish flesh, need close attention and inspection by the aquaculture industry and our government. Grocery stores and restaurants need to provide consumers with information as to where various seafood came from—ideally which ocean or which country or region of aquaculture (fish farm) production.

The worldwide community needs international conventions and enforcement of laws to save the oceans. Governments can help save the oceans, but none can make seafood safe for consumers in the foreseeable future. We must limit ocean fishing primarily to subsistence fishing for native peoples. Commercial fishing should be limited by strict quotas and net-size regulations. The conventional commercial fishing industry is neither sustainable nor ethical.

Aquaculture, a seemingly good solution for more fish protein, will not work unless it is organic and ecologically integrated with other farming practices. Aquabusiness factories raise seafood in a virtual soup of pharmaceuticals or from the open sewers and toxic waste dump sites that were once healthy oceans, rivers, and lakes. Most seafoods, touted as health food, clearly are not. Like much of the produce from livestock factory farms, the less of it we eat, the healthier we will be.

* * *

The oceans, which cover more than 70 percent of the earth's surface, are a vital source of food for a growing human population. The oceans also help stabilize and maintain our primary life-support system, the atmosphere. If we do not restore and protect the ocean ecosystems the problem of human hunger will pale before the global disruptions in climate that will follow the ecological collapse of the marine ecosystem. The restoration and protection of the oceans must be done for the good of the earth as a whole.

Chapter Six

Beware: You Are What You Eat

The cattle of the rich steal the bread of the poor.

Mohandas Gandhi

Our worldwide human population is now about 5.3 billion people. This is expected to double within two decades. Today, 28 percent of humans are malnourished. In order to meet the anticipated public demand for meat, we will have to at least double our current livestock population of some four and one-half billion animals. However, any increase in the current livestock population in order to feed this growing world population will come at a great cost to the natural world, and to the poor and hungry.

In the United States alone, the number of animals killed for food reached an all time high in 1995. According to the USDA's National Agricultural Statistics Services, this figure included 159 million cattle and calves, pigs, and sheep, as well as 8.68 billion chickens and turkeys.

Since the beginning of recorded history, most human communities, with few exceptions, killed animals for food. There were various restrictions and taboos, and those people who hunted, raised, and killed animals for food were not insensitive to the feelings of their prey. When our ancestors ate a meal, it was an act of communion. But in contemporary society, we have become so far removed from the land and the animals that sustain us that eating has become just another act of perfunctory consumption.

Most consumers never think to question where their meat came from, how the animals were treated while being raised, and how they were slaughtered. It is amazing that so many people will eat the parts and products of animals that have knowingly been caused to suffer prior to ending up on a fork. It is even more disturbing that so many people are unaware of or have never even thought about the creatures they eat.

When I used to eat meat, I accepted the animals' deaths as their inevitable, natural fate. And before I was aware of the severity of their unnecessary and unnatural suffering on factory farms and feedlots, I accepted meat—at least lean, well-cooked meat—with the same equanimity as I did vegetables, fruits, eggs, and dairy products. I used to think, "Food is food and meat is meat." I was raised to accept it without question or concern as to where it came from and how the creatures it came from were treated. I now avoid eating "anything that eats and had a mother."

The Dangers of Eating Meat

Aside from the ethical concerns, humans are not biologically suited nor physiologically adapted for a diet high in animal fat and protein. This kind of diet means that we eat proportionately less of important plant nutrients and suffer the consequences: developing a host of chronic degenerative diseases and faster aging.

Unfortunately, meat consumption is increasing in countries where, traditionally, plant-based diets were once predominant. There is an increased use and expansion of crop land in the United States to raise livestock feed for export since many Asian countries, such as China, are adopting a Western diet and can now afford to purchase more meat.

A widely held belief in Western society is that meat is more important for our health than foods of vegetable origin. However, the reverse is closer to the truth. All factory-farmed beef, pork and poultry meat, even with the surface fat and skin removed, are still high in saturated fat. In turn, this is converted by our livers into cholesterol. The lean portions of meat and poultry, eggs, and shrimp and lobster are all high in cholesterol. A high fat and cholesterol diet, combined with meat's high iron intake, is the prescription for atherosclerosis, heart attacks, strokes, and certain cancers. Diets high in animal protein are also linked with osteoporosis, gout, and increased susceptibility to gall bladder and kidney disease, among other illnesses.

In the more developed nations, where per capita meat consumption is higher than in poorer countries, there is a greater incidence of colon cancer and death from heart attacks and arteriosclerosis. Likewise, a correlation exists demographically between daily per capita intake of animal fat and death from breast cancer. Yet another cancer connection was found with meat in a 1996 study at the University of Iowa of women aged fifty-five to sixty-nine. Consumption of red meat—particularly hamburger—was associated with increased risk of non-Hodgkins lymphoma.

As for older people, it has been found that regular meat eaters are twice as likely as vegetarians to develop senile dementia. There might be a connection between pesticides and Alzheimer's disease, one of America's top three most debilitating and costly health problems in the elderly.[1]

An extensive study by the National Cancer Institute reveals a clear linkage between high-fat consumption and lung cancer.[2] Nonsmoking women with diets high in saturated fats had about four times the usual rate of lung cancer than those who ate more fruits and vegetables and less fat. Another study by the Wisconsin Medical School in Madison concluded that diets high in saturated fats and cholesterol raised the risk by 8 percent for the elderly who are prone to macular degeneration, a type of blindness. Simply by changing dietary habits to low-fat, low-cholesterol diets, most of these diseases are preventable.

The relatively low cost of food in the United States compared to other countries, coupled with increasingly sedentary lifestyles, is responsible for an alarming finding. One in three American adults is now seriously overweight, and the average body weight is increasing. This translates into fifty-eight million people being at increased risk from heart disease, diabetes, cancer, and other chronic ailments. The United States boasts a weight-loss industry that reaps $40 billion per year from American consumers. This is more than most countries spend on food.[3] Paradoxically, at the same time, the U.S. food industry spends some $36 billion a year on advertising processed food, which significantly contributes to weight gain.

The processed-food industry perpetuates our national high-calorie diet with prepared and processed convenience foods and relatively meaningless labeling of ingredient and daily recommended nutrient allowances. The poor American diet goes hand in hand with the over-consumptive and mal-consumptive (and malcontent) American society that justifies health spas, costly coronary bypasses, and liposuctions. In the meantime, the rest of the human population that might well aspire to live like those in Western civilization suffers from malnutrition and even starvation due in part to the insatiable appetites of the industrial world. Agricultural scientist Paul E. Waggoner observes:

> Today farmers feed five to six billion people by cultivating about a tenth of the planet's land. The seemingly irresistible doubling of population and the imperative of producing food will take another tenth of the land. Most of this land will come from Nature. This assumes people keep on eating and farmers keep on farming as they do now. So, farmers work at the junction where population, the human condition, and sparing land for Nature meet.[4]

Poisoned and Contaminated Meat

In late 1994, Gail Eisnitz, chief investigator for the California-based Humane Farming Association, blew the lid off a major meat scandal. She documented the routine sale of veal calves at slaughterhouses in the United States that had been treated with illegal, growth-boosting synthetic steroids. One of these drugs, clenbuterol—a beta agonist drug designed to stimulate unnatural rapid growth in livestock—is acutely poisonous to humans and has been implicated in the emergency hospitalizations of hundreds of Europeans who consumed contaminated veal calves' liver. People have gone into respiratory arrest from as little as one hamburger tainted with clenbuterol. Cooking has little effect on clenbuterol. "You have to virtually incinerate it," stated Lester Crawford, D.V.M., at a meeting of the Institute of Food Technologists. As long as the meat is edible by traditional standards, the clenbuterol is unaffected. In its pure form, just trace amounts of clenbuterol can cause nausea, dizziness, heart attack-like symptoms, breathing interruptions, and even death.

Eisnitz also uncovered documentation that revealed that the U.S. federal government secretly had been investigating leading veal companies across the country but withheld its findings from the public. Among those veal companies investigated was Wisconsin-based Provimi Veal Corporation, one of the nation's largest veal suppliers. Eisnitz turned over information to the media about the covert federal investigation. She then obtained eyeballs and bladders from veal calves at U.S. slaughterhouses and sent them to the world's foremost clenbuterol testing facility in The Netherlands for independent testing. The results revealed that the U.S. veal supply was laden with clenbuterol.

In June 1996, Vitek Supply Corporation, the nation's leading veal feed supplement manufacturer, and its president, Jannes Doppenberg, were both convicted of distributing more than 1.7 million pounds of tainted feed. They were found guilty on twelve felony counts each of smuggling and distributing drug-tainted feed to at least eleven leading veal companies in the United States.[5]

In January 1997, Doppenberg was sentenced to serve a forty-four-month prison term. Both Doppenberg and Vitek Supply Corporation were ordered to pay fines and restitution totaling more than $1 million.[6] The Vitek conviction is considered to be the tip of the iceberg in regard to the veal industry's use of this deadly drug. The U.S. Department of Justice has publicly vowed to prosecute several other leading veal companies in connection with this case.[7] (See endnote for further developments in this veal investigation.)

The use of clenbuterol in livestock to produce leaner carcasses, although illegal, raises serious concerns for public health and safety. In February 1995, a Belgian veterinarian, Dr. Karel Van Noppen, who was investigating the illegal use of hormones by some European livestock producers, was shot to death by the "hormone mafia," the organized crime network of illegal animal drug dealers. Soon after the shooting, the European Parliament (Belgium, Denmark, Germany, France, Italy, Ireland, Luxembourg, The Netherlands, and the United Kingdom) voted unanimously in favor of a resolution calling for the end of the use of growth hormones in livestock. Health experts from France were especially concerned about children who ate veal on a regular basis, because boys were developing breasts and girls were developing large clitorides.

Crawford promised that the Food Safety Inspection Service (FSIS) will now conduct an exploratory program for clenbuterol and other beta agonists in a variety of animals. He added that the FSIS would also like to start a new heavy-metal survey, which will look largely for lead, cadmium, and mercury.

Fraud and disregard for consumer health and safety continue to blight agribusiness' meat industry sector. For instance, federal agents in Oakland, California, seized one hundred thousand pounds of sausage made from cattle that inspectors had previously labeled 4-D: diseased, disabled, down, and dying.[8] United States military bases inadvertently purchased 75 percent of the tainted sausage. Federal law prohibits 4-D meat from human consumption; however, it usually ends up in pet food, fertilizer, or livestock and poultry feed.[9]

Farm animal and consumer health concerns over the safety of 4-D meat continue to be an unresolved issue. Veterinarian Leslie P. Williams, Jr. voices legitimate concern that manufacturers should not use 4-D meat at all, in a raw state, for animal feeding.[9] In his studies, dogs got sick from *Salmonella* bacteria when fed 4-D meat from rendering plants. Some dogs that did not become sick became carriers of *Salmonella*, excreting the bacteria in their feces. *E. coli* bacteria in the intestines of these test dogs even acquired antibiotic resistance from these *Salmonella* bacteria that were highly resistant to antibiotics.

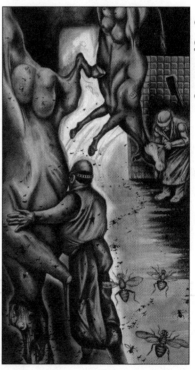

Courtesy of Sue Coe

Children in the United States who regularly consume hot dogs more than once a week have twice the risk of developing leukemia according to P. Giem, M.D., and co-workers.[10] Their risk of developing brain tumors doubles if their mothers ate hot dogs and other processed meats during pregnancy. Nitrates are blamed. Processors use nitrate as a preservative. During cooking, the nitrate becomes overheated and converts into harmful nitrosamine.

The earlier onset of puberty in girls and boys on a Western meat-based diet also reflects the profound effect that animal fat and hormones in our food can have on human development. Substances implanted in beef cattle to make them grow faster include trenbolone acetate, a synthetic testosterone, and zeranol, a synthetic estrogen, and are widely used. Also, a widely used group of pesticides called organochlorines, which persist in the environment and become concentrated in animal fat and human mothers' milk, have recently been found to mimic estrogens (along with dioxins) in the human body. Ionophores, beta blockers and beta agonists are some of the newer so-called "smart" drugs used by the beef, pork, and veal industries to boost growth. Little is known of their safety for consumers. Some, like clenbuterol, are very harmful and are used illegally.

People with compromised immune systems from diseases such as cancer, AIDS, diabetes, or developing fetuses and nursing infants, organ-graft recipients, and allergy sufferers are at risk when they eat meat. Due to their impaired immune systems, they are more prone to bacterial food poisoning. Federal government health experts advise people who are on antibiotics not to eat hamburger.

In 1989 the U.S. Department of Agriculture issued a mandate ordering McDonalds and other hamburger food chains to cook all meat thoroughly. Medium-and rare-cooked hamburger is a health hazard. Ironically, cooking meat is also a health hazard, since cancer-causing fumes and residues in the meat rise from burned fat.

In order to protect against bacterially contaminated meat, agribusiness entrepreneurs are pushing for meat irradiation. However, a recent research study raises grave doubts over the effectiveness of irradiation to prevent bacterial contamination of poultry.[11] Irradiation does kill *Salmonella*, a common cause of food poisoning. Unfortunately, it also kills beneficial bacteria over the surface of deboned chicken meat. Some of these beneficial bacteria have the capacity to slow the growth of *Salmonella* and other harmful bacteria. If the irradiated meat becomes re-contaminated with *Salmonella* or any other bacteria (a frequent occurrence in contaminated processing facilities), the harmful bacteria will be able to spread rapidly, thereby undoing any purported benefit of the initial irradiation.

Milk Risks

Our ancestors gave their children milk from cows that grazed on fresh forages of green pastures. Today, the modern dairy cow on a factory farm produces so much milk that she can weaken and succumb to foot and udder infections. Bacteria are a dairy farmer's worst enemy because they can contaminate milk and make cows sick. Farmers use a host of antibiotics to treat these disorders. (See Chapter Two for a detailed discussion.) However, the Food and Drug Administration (FDA) is unable to effectively detect and regulate drug residues in our milk supply.[12] Astonishingly, the FDA, under industry pressure, has approved the use of genetically engineered bovine growth hormone (rBGH) injections to make cows produce even more milk. In doing this, the FDA has completely ignored studies that show cows treated with rBGH have a higher incidence of lameness and mastitis.[13] This higher incidence of infection means farmers will use even more antibiotics —and milk could be even more of a health risk. (See Chapter Four on rBGH.)

There is a myth fostered by the American Dairy Association that says children and adults must have plenty of milk to obtain calcium for strong bones and teeth. In truth, vegetables such as broccoli and kale provide plenty of calcium that children are better able to absorb than the calcium in cow's milk. The high protein content of milk (and of a diet high in animal protein) actually increases calcium loss in the urine by interfering with calcium absorption in the digestive tract.[14]

Milk consumption may play a role in such debilitating diseases as migraine, arthritis, infant colic, diabetes, and cataracts. Doctors often diagnose lactose intolerance and allergic reactions to cow's milk, including asthma, headaches, diarrhea, and fatigue. This points to yet another hazard to both children and adults. Nursing mothers who consume dairy products can pass on various milk proteins of bovine origin in their milk. Their infants may then develop colic.[15] According to R.R. Coombs and S.T. Holgate, through mother's milk, infants can become sensitized to bovine milk proteins and develop an acute allergic reaction that may result in sudden infant death syndrome.[16]

Researchers in Canada and Finland have recently implicated cow's milk in the development of juvenile diabetes.[17] Infants who are genetically susceptible to diabetes should not drink cow's milk. Whey protein, called bovine serum albumen, causes these children to produce antibodies against the whey protein and a similar protein in the cells of the pancreas that produce insulin. This reaction destroys the insulin-producing cells, thus creating a diabetic condition. The findings of this research may explain why the incidence of diabetes parallels the per capita consumption of milk in various countries. It may also corroborate the finding that breast-fed babies are less likely to become diabetic than those fed a formula containing cow's milk.

The well-documented link between consumption of cow's milk and the development of juvenile diabetes[18] is not the only health problem that can arise from feeding cow's milk to infants.[19] The American Academy of Pediatrics recommends not to give cow's milk to infants under twelve months of age because it may cause iron deficiency anemia.[20] This is not because milk is low in iron but because bovine albumin in the milk can cause an immune reaction in the intestinal tract, which leads to blood loss from the intestinal tract.[21]

Food and Our Emotions

We do not yet fully know what chemicals in our foods do to our minds and bodies. However, the neurological, developmental, psychological, immunological, sexual, and behavioral changes that have been found in animals (both in the wild and in laboratory tests) as a result of having some of these chemicals injected or put in their food and water are alarming.

It is well known that a high level of the sex hormone testosterone in the blood of adolescents are associated with a greater incidence of aggressive-destructive behavior, impatience, and irritability.[22] A diet high in animal fat and low in fiber leads to a retention of sex hormones in the body. However, the plant fiber of vegetables binds circulating hormones excreted in the bile from the liver, preventing their re-uptake in the small intestine. A high plant diet elevates the amount of sex hormone binding globulin (SHBG) in the blood.[23, 24] Neal Barnard, M.D., in his book *Eat Right, Live Longer*, explains:

> **SHBG is a protein molecule which acts like an aircraft carrier that holds the estrogen or testosterone "airplanes" until they are needed. It keeps sex hormones in check. The result is not only a more stable menstrual cycle or reduced cancer risk. The psyche seems to be affected as well. In the Massachusetts Male Aging Study, a large, ongoing study of middle-aged and older men in the Boston area, researchers have found that those men with more SHBG in their blood are less domineering and aggressive. It may well be that a better diet can make you (or bring you) an easier-to-get-along-with partner.[25]**

Since sex hormones can have a profound affect on our mood and behavior,[26] we should be mindful of the fact that a diet high in animal fat—including dairy products that contain traces of bovine estrogen—will disrupt our hormonal balance. When we become obese, our own body fat manufactures estrogen, further compounding the effects of a meat-based, high-fat diet. Impotence and infertility, prostate cancer in meat-based, high-fat diet. Impotence and infertility, prostate cancer in males, and breast cancer and distressingly difficult menopause in women can be curbed by a change in diet.

In addition, how animals are slaughtered can affect their carcasses' chemical makeup, which in turn can affect the systems of those who eat them. Our ancestors never consumed animals that had been subjected to the stress and terror of being loaded and trucked long distances for many hours to slaughter plants, then made to wait in fear, often suffering great exhaustion, thirst, hunger, and painful injuries before they are killed. Most often these animals experience additional stress while witnessing other animals struggling and thrashing as they are slaughtered. Studies show that animals stressed prior to slaughter have a higher lactic acid content in their meat, and the texture of the meat also changes. Stress in pigs results in "PSE" (pale- soft-exudative) meat, and in dry "dark cutters" in beef carcasses. Meat from animals terrified prior to slaughter could affect consumers' mood and behavior.

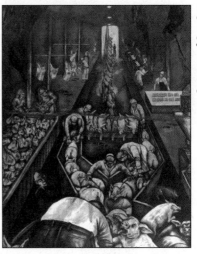

Courtsey of Sue Coe

In the past, animals for food were either killed swiftly by skilled hunters or else they were killed quickly, not in a fearful, stressful state by the people they knew on the farm. Meat eaters knew that the flesh of stressed animals would quickly spoil. The Native American's advice to a novice hunter was: "Kill the deer swiftly with one arrow, otherwise you will feed its fear to your family."

It is highly probable that the biochemistry of stressed animals, especially the steroid stress hormones present in their flesh, has an effect on the behavior and metabolism of consumers. Animals who have been subjected to violence and terror may pass on the biochemical products of these psychosomatic reactions in their various bodily parts, which people consume. Considering the tons of such adulterated flesh consumed in a lifetime, the psychological effects may well be cumulative and may profoundly influence mood and behavior, especially in the realms of violence, anxiety disorders, and sexual and social development. This possibility warrants further study, considering the well-documented adverse physical effects of high-meat consumption on the human body.

There are few studies evaluating mood or personality changes following dietary change, such as changing from a meat to plant-based diet. Anecdotal evidence suggests that people who do not eat meat have a calmer, more easy-going disposition. One carefully controlled study reported in the British medical journal, *The Lancet*,[27] lends some support to such anecdotal evidence. F.G.R. Fowkes, M.D., and associates discovered that serum triglyceride concentration (especially in men) relates to hostile acts and domineering attitude. They found lower concentrations in more easygoing nonmeat eaters.

Also disturbing are the social consequences of institutionalized violence towards animals during the mass slaughter of millions of animals every week in the United States. Animal factory farms and feedlots condone and institutionalize violence to animals on the grounds of economics and "efficiency." The spiral of violence created by this industrial process also includes the obliteration of rural communities and sustainable, humane, and nature-friendly farming practices, along with the annihilation of wildlife and their habitats.

Compassionate Kitchens

Just as we concern ourselves with ending domestic violence among humans, we must also consider the violence people bring into their kitchens when they purchase animal products from factory farms. I believe that more compassionate kitchens would result in less violent households.

The violence in contemporary society will not be extinguished so long as violence toward animals continues to be accepted as "normal." If we do not change our diets out of protest, as well as for our own physical and psychological well-being, large-scale violence towards animals will continue to increase as the world's appetite increases for meat.

The first and most significant and beneficial step we can all take is to change our diets. Consumers, one by one, can contribute toward changing the market-driven system that sustains large agribusiness products, such as pesticides, antibiotics, growth hormones, and synthetic fertilizers. If consumers insisted that grocery stores carry certified organic produce, this would encourage farmers and ranchers, as well as food processors, wholesalers and retailers, to support and empower a more sustainable farming culture. Another simple but powerful consumer action would be to eliminate a meat-based meal a few times a week, and buy only meat that is humanely grown, such as free-range chickens, which are free of hormones and antibiotics.

The future of agriculture depends upon a reawakening of this empathic realm of being in the world, which is implicit in the term "husbandry." This includes the future well-being of farm animals, the land, and nature's resources. To husband implies a kind of marriage based upon respect, understanding and feeling for animals, plants, and the good earth itself. Empathic husbandry is the heart of a sustainable agriculture and the key to a sustainable future.

These kinds of consumer choices would soon influence farming practices. In the final analysis, *it is not what comes out of our mouths that will make any difference; rather, it is what we choose to put into our mouths.*

Chapter Seven

Power of the Plate:
Eating for a Greener World

The ultimate goal of farming is not the growing of crops but the cultivation and perfection of human beings.

Masanobu Fukuoka, farmer-philosopher

E ach individual can make a difference in creating a greener world. Every meal choice can move us one step closer to a more sustainable agriculture, and ultimately, healthier lives. By simply cutting down on the amount of meat eaten in one week, each consumer can begin to have a long-term impact, personally as well as globally.

In the 1990s the food industry has seen a marked shift in consumers' diets, turning away from high-volume meat consumption. This shift was recognized by the National Restaurant Association, which in turn urged its one hundred fifty thousand members to offer vegetarian sections on their menus. A nationwide Gallup poll found that one out of every five restaurant goers seeks out eateries serving vegetarian food, and one out of every three consumers will order nonmeat dishes if available.[1] In turn, the beef industry upped its pro-meat advertising campaign declaring, beef is "real food for real people." Pork producers also found a new angle to appeal to consumers' new consciousness about avoiding "red meat." They declared that pork is "the other white meat," along with chicken.

Together, consumers and farmers must make fundamental changes in attitude and conscience. The challenge to farm with less harm entails more than a change in agricultural systems, technologies, and policies. Albert Einstein wisely surmised: "The significant problems of the world cannot be solved at the same level of consciousness at which they were created."

For humans, eating was once a sacred act of communion, for sustenance of the body, as well as for the mind and soul. The good farmer, provider of wholesome food, steward of the land, held the respect of consumers. But today, as we move into the twenty-first century, we have an excessive abundance of unnatural, unsafe, and costly foods. We process, freeze, dehydrate, irradiate, pasteurize, convenience, junk, snack, microwave, vacuum-pack, enrich, and even laboratory-create food. Western society already has highly automated, almost farmerless farms producing the raw materials that processors mix with synthetic ingredients to provide consumers with this variety of unnatural foods.

Spokespeople for the agribusiness food industry claim to only cater to public taste and give the public "what they want." Supposedly the public wants a cheap and plentiful supply of food. The economic and health problems created by overproduction and overconsumption are a chronic consequence of a highly technical and highly competitive market system.

With the advent of advanced food technologies, particularly genetic engineering biotechnology, the next generation may well encounter a marketplace almost devoid of natural food. Instead, there will be a host of synthetic food manufactured entirely in the laboratories of a few mega-corporations that dominate the industry. "Real food is for real people" and "We are what we eat"—No truer words have ever been spoken; nor have these sayings had such an important message as they do today.

Less Meat, More Plants

Some livestock producers will criticize this book because it promotes eating less meat, and if possible, vegetarianism. There will also be vegetarians who will be unhappy because I do not promote vegetarianism exclusively. Instead, I advocate eating with conscience, which may include eating animal products. I realize that consumers must make their own informed dietary choices, and that what may work well for one individual may not work for another. I have argued many times for vegetarianism; however, I also recognize that this must be presented as a personal choice and not as dogma. Vegetarianism is one option for living gently and being a conscientious consumer.

Eating some meat and poultry is acceptable, especially for those

Food for Thought

♦ Calories and protein equally distributed from present crop land could give a vegetarian diet to ten billion people;

♦ The global totals of sun on land, carbon dioxide in the air, fertilizer, and even water could produce far more food than ten billion people need;

♦ By eating different species of crops, and mostly vegetarian diets, we can change the number who can be fed from a plot;

♦ Millions of people do change their diets in response to health, price, and other pressures, and that they are capable of changing their diet even further;

♦ Given adequate incentives, farmers can use new technologies to increase food productivity and thus keep prices level—despite a rising population. Even better use of existing technology can raise current yields;

♦ Despite recurring problems with water supply and distribution, there are opportunities to raise more crops with the same volume of water;

♦ In Europe and the United States, rising income, improving technology, and leveling populations forecast diminishing use of crop land.

By Paul E. Waggoner, agriculturalist, from: "How Much Land Can 10 Billion People Spare for Nature?" Monograph. Ames, Iowa: Council for Agriculture, Science, and Technology. 1994.

living in rural communities and who are directly responsible for humanely raising and slaughtering the animals they eat. The best meat, milk, and eggs come from livestock and poultry who are free to roam, eat organic feed, and live in an environment that satisfies their basic behavioral requirements. A growing number of farmers and ranchers are working for better ways to care for the land and to treat their animals with respect and compassion.

From my perspective as an animal welfare reformer, the most crucial concern is that consumers make choices that help keep farmers on

the land and keep the corporations out. When consumers support ecologically conscious livestock farmers, they are supporting sustainable
agriculture. This means not purchasing any animal products that come
from the agribusiness conglomerates that have contracted with "growers" to operate factory farms. It is not enough simply to conscientious-
ly reduce consumption of animal products from inhumane farming
systems, it also means consumers need to actively support humane and
organic farmers with their buying power. This could be as simple as
buying eggs laid by "free-ranging, drug-free" hens. Not only are you
improving your health, but you are supporting farmers who humanely
raise their birds. What if consumers across the country insisted that
major supermarket chains offer the choice of hormone-free, free-ranging chickens, and eggs from uncaged hens? This alone would be revolutionary!

A powerful step for caring consumers is to choose a humane diet
that reduces or eliminates meat. Choosing a humane diet is a powerful
consumer action to prevent and reverse further loss of biodiversity and
natural resources. Choosing a humane diet also helps alleviate the need
for factory farms simply because it reduces consumer demand for meat.

The least ecologically damaging, humane, and sustainable diet is
not meat-based, but plant-based and organic. There are several kinds of
vegetarians. They include *lacto-ovo-vegetarians*, the most common vegetarians in the United States, who do not eat meat, poultry, fish, or
seafood, but do consume milk, milk products, and eggs. A *lacto-vegetar-
ian* is similar, but excludes eggs. *Piscitarians* are fish-eating vegetarians. *Vegans* (pronounced VEE-gun) avoid all animal products, including
dairy, eggs, and possibly honey. Vegans may even refuse to wear leather, silk, fur, or wool, based on a philosophy that each sentient animal
has a right to his or her body and life.

People decide to cut back on meat or stop eating meat for a variety
of reasons. As someone who has worked in animal welfare for more
than twenty years, I decided to not eat meat for three major reasons:

+ **The welfare of intensively raised farm animals;**

+ **The impact of the intensive livestock industry on wildlife
   and natural habitat;**

+ **The demise of family farms and rural communities, largely due
   to the expansion of conventional industrial farming systems.**

My grown daughter, Camilla, who works in animal welfare, became a vegetarian long before I did, and my other daughter, Mara, who is now thirteen years old, decided when she was four that she would not eat animals. At the time, she reasoned, "If people can eat animals, then animals should be able to eat people. Now that's wrong, so I don't want to eat animals."

When consumers buy with more compassion for animals and the environment, they are encouraging farmers to farm with less harm. This kind of consumer involvement will lead to a reduction in the production and consumption of meat overall, and ultimately, an incentive for more and more farmers to improve their farming. These kinds of choices also contribute to a healthier and longer life.

The Natural Diet

People who insist that it is natural for us to eat meat, poultry, seafood, eggs, and dairy produce are only partially correct. First, most of these products are neither natural nor healthy anymore. Second, our gatherer-hunter ancestors were attuned to a diet that was, for most ethnic groups, very low in animal fat and protein. Wild animals are mostly lean and lacking in saturated fats, unlike the fat feedlot cattle, pigs, and factory poultry that people consume today. Many of the mental and physical health problems today are linked with improper diets that are not suitable for us physiologically. During 99 percent of our time on earth as *Homo sapiens*, our diet was that of the gatherer-hunter, and primarily plant-based.

Human physiology has not changed significantly since the advent of agriculture some eight to ten thousand years ago. Humans are still a plant-dependent animal. Our bodies do not make vitamin C, and we rely on plants for this vital nutrient as well as for other nutrients such as riboflavin, beta carotenoids, calcium, iron, selenium, magnesium, boron, and zinc. Plants give us soluble fiber, an important dietary component absent in animal products. Fiber helps rid the body of toxins and hormones and prevents their reabsorption in the intestines. And plant fiber also helps lower blood cholesterol and triglyceride levels that are linked with atherosclerosis and heart attacks.

We rely on a plant-based diet to help our cells deal with the potentially carcinogenic effects of free radicals that are produced in our bodies increasingly as we age. Free radicals are neutralized by oxidants like vitamins C, and E, and selenium. Beta carotenes help the immune system by stimulating the production of white blood cells ("killer" cells and T-helper cells). Facts such as these demonstrate how incredibly dependent our bodies are upon various plant nutrients and "nutriceuticals" in order to maintain health and to cope with stress. Equally nutritious, and in many aspects more healthful, protein substitutes of vegetable origin are viable alternatives to animal products.

One of the reasons why there is a linkage between low polyunsaturated fat consumption and heart disease is because we do not eat enough leafy greens. Furthermore, conventionally raised farm animals cannot graze on beneficial wild plants. Therefore, their diets are generally lacking in polyunsaturated fatty acids. R.W. Lacey, M.D., says, "Changes in the methods of feeding food animals, poultry and fish, and their processing, may be partly responsible for the continued high incidence of coronary heart disease."[2]

In July 1992, the United States National Cancer Institute (NCI) launched 5-A Day for Better Health, a nationwide, five-year campaign to encourage Americans to eat more daily servings of fruits and vegetables. This was a joint effort between the NCI and the Produce for Better Health Foundation, an organization established by the fruit and vegetable industry. In addition, the American Cancer Society confirmed there is a lower incidence of colon cancer in people who include a variety of vegetables, fruits, and grains in their diets.[3] A long-term study of diet and health in Germany concluded that vegetarians experienced one-third of the deaths expected from heart disease. They also experienced only half of the deaths and diseases linked to respiratory and digestive system disorders.[4]

In recent studies on caloric intake and aging at the University of Wisconsin, researchers found that the muscles of old rats were similar to those of much younger rats when they were given a diet low in calories. Richard Weindruch, M.D., believes the results strengthen a theory that says aging is the result of biological damage inflicted by oxygen molecules called "free radicals." These highly reactive oxygen molecules are a natural byproduct of metabolism, and are produced by the body in quantities proportional to the amount of food consumed. These findings support the theory that muscle and other cells are spared the damaging effects of free radicals when we don't overeat. The more we eat, the more free radicals are produced as a natural byproduct of metabolism.[5]

USDA Food Guide Pyramid

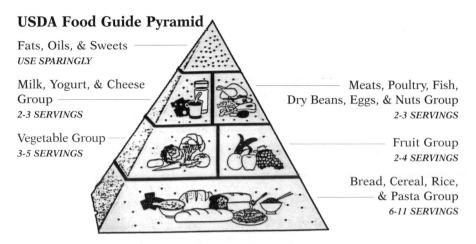

Fats, Oils, & Sweets
USE SPARINGLY

Milk, Yogurt, & Cheese Group
2-3 SERVINGS

Meats, Poultry, Fish, Dry Beans, Eggs, & Nuts Group
2-3 SERVINGS

Vegetable Group
3-5 SERVINGS

Fruit Group
2-4 SERVINGS

Bread, Cereal, Rice, & Pasta Group
6-11 SERVINGS

Eating Wrong with USDA Recommendations

The Four Basic Food Groups that the United States Department of Agriculture has promoted for decades recommends that people eat equal servings per day from the Meat, Dairy and Egg, Fruit and Vegetable, and Bread-Cereal groups. This USDA food wheel includes high-protein legumes and nuts under its "meat group."

In the USDA's new Food Guide Pyramid there are five food groups—that includes "Fats, Oils, and Sweets." The new pyramid recommends proportionately more servings from the Bread-Cereal group than in the previous guide. The USDA is recommending that about one-third of a person's daily diet should be animal fat and protein. Beans and nuts still remain in the meat category. It is odd and biologically inconsistent that the USDA places beans and nuts in the meat, fish, poultry, and egg category. Dairy foods of comparable protein value, for example, are in a separate category.

In my opinion, the new Food Guide Pyramid regimen of the USDA is an "Eating Wrong" proposal that encourages conspicuous consumption. Harvard University medical nutrition expert, Walter C. Willett, M.D., cautions:

> The U.S. food industry is responding rapidly to widespread concerns about diet and health, primarily with an array of new low-fat products. However, many of these products have substituted the fat with sugar, diglycerides (which do not count as fat on food labels), artificial sweeteners, and sucrose polyesters. In addition, there has been an increase in consumption of lean meat.[6]

Pyramid Food Guide
for a Humane and Healthy Life and Planet

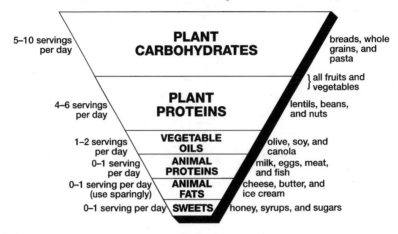

The implicit recommendation from the USDA is that consumers should avoid fat. It is absurd then, that they should get most of their protein from fat-laden animal sources—meat, eggs, and dairy products. It is even more absurd to suggest these fatty products should make up about one-third of our diet. This is way beyond the protein requirements of normal healthy adults who will simply excrete the excess protein. Much of this protein goes to supply the body with energy that can be more readily and cheaply obtained from vegetable oils and carbohydrates.

Beans and nuts will satisfy our protein needs just as well as eggs, meat, poultry, and dairy products. Vegetable proteins, such as dry beans, peas, nuts, and seeds are far more energy and farm-labor efficient than animal protein, and environmentally easier to store. Also, animal fat turns rancid faster than vegetable oils. An energy-conscious society, therefore, looks for alternatives to the need to refrigerate, or irradiate most of the foods. Such a society follows the wisdom of its agrarian ancestors.

A diet based on these recommendations might look more like the one depicted in the inverted pyramid above, which supports good health as well as sustainable farming. It also meets daily trace mineral and vitamin requirements.

Researchers T. Colin Campbell and Chen Junshi reported a surprising finding following their comprehensive comparative study of dietary, lifestyle, and health differences in China and more industrialized Western societies. The study reported: "Even small intakes of foods of

Western Diseases of Known and Possible Dietary Origin

Autoimmune Diseases - Diabetes (type I or insulin dependent), autoimmune thyroiditis.

Cancer - Colorectal, breast, prostate, lung, endometrium, ovarian.

Cardiovascular - Coronary heart disease, cerebrovascular disease, (stroke), essential hypertension, deep vein thrombosis, pulmonary embolism, pelvic phleboliths, varicose veins.

Gastrointestinal - Constipation, hiatus hernia, appendicitis, diverticular disease, colorectal polyps, Crohn's disease (regional ileitis), celiac disease, peptic ulcer, hemorrhoids, ulcerative colitis.

Metabolic - Obesity, diabetes (type II or noninsulin dependent), cholesterol gallstones, renal stones, osteoporosis, gout.

Other Disorders - Allergies, immunoinsufficiency, infantile hyperactivity, migraine, multiple sclerosis, pernicious anemia, rheumatoid arthritis, spina bifida, thyrotoxicosis.

Modified after D.P. Burkitt in *Western Diseases: Their Dietary Prevention and Reversibility.* N.J. Temple and D.P. Burkitt (eds). Totowa, New Jersey. Humana Press. 1994.

animal origin are associated with significant increases in plasma cholesterol concentrations, which are associated, in turn, with significant increases in chronic degenerative disease mortality rates." [7]

It is irresponsible for the United States government to continue not to inform the public *fully* about the environmental and health costs of a meat-based diet. However, to do so may not be politically prudent, but not to do so is unethical. As Neal Barnard, M.D., observes in his book *Food for Life*:

> The traditional four food groups and the eating patterns they prescribe have led to cancer and heart disease in epidemic numbers, and have killed more people than any other factor in America. More than automobile accidents, more than tobacco, more than all the wars of this century combined.[8]

Foods That Heal

From the perspectives of natural farming, natural health, and natural diet, Japanese farmer-philosopher Masanobu Fukuoka states, "Meat is yang, vegetables yin, with grains in between. Because man is an omnivorous animal that is yang. This leads to a set of principles that says that when grains, which are intermediate, are eaten as a staple, yin vegetables should be consumed. And meat (very yang)—consumption of which is essentially cannibalism—should be avoided."[9]

Humans are a highly adaptable primate species. One feature of our adaptive success is our capacity to be omnivorous. We have the flexibility to eat from a wide range of food sources, from fruits to nuts, and meats to maize. We have developed remarkable ways to preserve and enhance the nutritive value and palatability of a diversity of natural foods. Cultural and ethnic differences in cuisine reflect biogeographic and seasonal variations in food types and availability. This diversity provides a rich cornucopia of culinary delights and creates a demand for new crops and food products for an increasingly cosmopolitan marketplace.

From this cornucopia, we can select some of the most tried and true diets that have been tested for countless generations, and that are also ecologically sound and sustainable. One classic example, Mediterranean cuisine, integrates various foods to provide an extremely healthful, relatively low-cost, and ecologically sustainable diet.

For reasons of public health, economy, and corporate profitability, it would be smart for the food industry to develop more alternatives to red meat and poultry. Soyburgers, "Veggie Burgers," and "gardenburgers" are now popular meatless items in many supermarkets and restaurants. There are greater economic and energy savings to be realized from turning grains and legumes directly into human food rather than feeding them to animals to convert into marketable meat.

Vegetables and fruits are not only an excellent source of low-calorie nutrient energy, essential vitamins, minerals, and beneficial fiber, but they also contain other ingredients called phytochemicals that help prevent cancer and other chronic diseases. For example, genistein, which occurs in soy-based food, prevents the proliferation of cancer cells and of new blood vessels that make tumors grow.

Soybean products are especially promising in reducing cholesterol levels and certain cancers, especially breast cancer. Soybeans also contain phytoestrogens, which may help women during menopause because plant estrogen—like the soy component genistein—seem to block the harmful effects of human estrogen. Animal studies show that soybean protein helps prevent bone loss (osteoporosis) caused by ovarian hormone deficiency. Soybean products like tofu may therefore help create healthy bones by increasing bone density.[10] Soy protein actually mimics the effects of the anticancer drug tamoxifen.[11] Certain enzymes found in cabbage-like vegetables detoxify carcinogens. Food chemists have also identified natural antioxidants in various fruits and vegetables that deactivate free radicals that can damage DNA and cause cancer.

A group of compounds, the indole-3-carbinol conjugates—found in broccoli and related brassica vegetables—are also anti-estrogenic. These "nutriceuticals" or phytochemicals are important, especially in light of increased breast and testicular cancer, and other forms of cancer and fertility problems. These types of cancers are associated with exposure to dioxin, DDT, PCBs, and other organochlorine pesticides in the environment that have estrogenic properties and depress the immune system. Of course, the benefits of these and other plant products are likely to be less if they were not produced organically.

The field of food science is still in its infancy. Variables such as soil quality, plant variety, and how we raise and process cereals, fruits, and vegetables need more research to discover how these factors affect human nutrition. Yet research has already proven that fruits, herbs, vegetables, and cereals do have a vital role in disease prevention and perhaps in the aging process.

Even considering all the benefits fruits and vegetables provide, one must be careful to learn which foods are safest to eat. Foods such as carrots and concentrated juices are likely to have high levels of pesticides. Carrots absorb harmful chemicals present in the soil and have been used to help clean up contaminated soil. If at all possible, a consumer's safest choice is to buy organic products thereby avoiding chemical and pesticide exposure.

The National Cancer Institute (NCI) dedicates, on average, a mere 5 percent of its approximate annual budget of $1.8 billion to preventive medicine. The NCI spends much more on gene therapy and other biotechnology-based treatments. This certainly gives me pause for concern. Our efforts should be focused on prevention.

Nutritional Considerations

A $2.3 million study by Cornell University Professor Colin Campbell and associates compared the health and dietary habits of Americans with those of the Chinese who eat little meat, animal fat, and dairy products.[12] The results of the study show that Americans have a higher incidence of obesity, heart disease, cancer, and diabetes. High cancer rates, especially of the breast and reproductive organs, can result from childhood diets high in calories, protein, fat, and calcium that promote rapid growth. The study's director, T. Colin Campbell, a nutritional biochemist, states, "We are basically a vegetarian species and should be eating a wide variety of plant foods and minimizing our intake of animal foods." Dr. Campbell also emphasizes, "Usually the first thing a country does in the course of economic development is to introduce a lot of livestock. Our data are showing that this is not a very smart move."

This study also shows that we do not need meat to prevent iron-deficiency anemia or other conditions. Chinese consume twice the iron Americans do, their primary source being vegetables. Likewise, Hans-Michael Dosch, M.D., and coworkers contend on the basis of their research that it is a myth that cow's milk is an essential calcium source needed to prevent osteoporosis. In China, osteoporosis is rare. Most Chinese consume no dairy products, and instead get the calcium they need from vegetables.

This same study, led by Dr. Dosch, found that vegetarians have significantly lower standardized mortality ratios for all causes, and especially heart disease. In the study, the benefits of a vegetarian diet were quite independent of lifestyle, geography, and other factors such as weight, smoking, and social class.[13] These findings support a report in the *British Medical Journal* that states vegetarians are 40 percent less likely to die of cancer than meat eaters.[14]

The adequacy of vegetarian diets still concerns some health professionals and many consumers who have heard the myths surrounding vegetarian diets. However, the American Dietetic Association (ADA) has stated, "Vegetarian diets are healthful and nutritionally adequate when appropriately planned." Nutritionists T. Sanders and S. Reddy have shown that a properly selected vegetarian diet can meet all the requirements of adults and growing children.[15] A vegetarian diet takes education and planning, but it is not difficult to learn what foods fulfill what nutritional needs. For example, a few simple considerations, such as ensuring adequate iron, calcium, and vitamins D and B-12 intake can make a vegetarian diet nutritionally complete. There are numerous publications and books for vegetarians, who now number more than twelve million in the United States, according to a survey by *Vegetarian Times*. This is twice the number of vegetarians as there were in 1985.[16]

Plant-Based Solutions

A potential treasure trove of invaluable plant varieties awaits discovery and immediate protection. These plants exist in the oceans, forests, meadows, savannas, swamps, and bushland of every nation. Significantly, the preservation of natural biodiversity, coupled with documentation of indigenous medical knowledge, may be one of the wisest choices of this millennium.

Presently, distributors of plant-based supplements cannot print any medical claims on the product label. The FDA insists on this to deter quacks and charlatans, and to that extent it is a useful law. However, there are many plant-based medications that are excellent remedies, and usually at a fraction of the cost of traditional medicine. Unfortunately, the only way for people to learn about beneficial plant-based products is through word-of-mouth or from publications outside mainstream nutrition and medicine. This is hardly a suitable way to inform millions of people of the benefits of individual plant-based supplements.

Conventional medicine's current indifference toward research and development in plant-based nutrient supplements and preventive and curative medications is indeed a backward step. There is great potential for legitimate and considerable corporate profits in this field, especially for farmers and horticulturists. Plant-based medications such as echinacea and supplements like zinc are not attractive to most corporations because they cannot patent them. Conversely, new-generation, genetically engineered products, like interferon, will be costly, but patentable and highly profitable. We are increasingly in need of new generation medicines to treat and prevent the rising number and variety of diseases among humans. The earth's plants hold many solutions, if only we would invest our money and time in plant research.

Potential Cancer Fighters in Foods

Although no food or food combination has yet been clinically proven to prevent or retard cancer in people, research strongly suggests that many components have specific biological actions that may prove helpful. Scientists suspect that to treat tumors, compounds would have to be extracted or synthesized and given in larger doses than those found naturally; on the other hand, extracts or synthesis might overlook protective compounds, in a healthful varied diet. The following list offers some food sources that may be beneficial for their possible desease-fighting properties.

Component	Possible disease-fighting properties	Food sources
Allylic sulfides	May protect against carcinogens by stimulating production of a detoxification enzyme, glutathione-S-transferase	Garlic and onion
Carotenoids, (Vitamin A precursors)	Antioxidants and cell differentiation agents (cancer cells are nondifferentiated)	Parsley, carrots, winter squash, sweet potatoes, yams, cantaloupe, apricots, spinach, kale, turnip greens, citrus fruits
Catechins (tannins)	Antioxidants, linked to lower rates of gastro-intestinal cancer; mechanisms not understood	Green tea, berries
Flavonoids	Block receptor sites for certain hormones that promote cancers	Most fruits and vegetables, including parsley, carrots, citrus fruits, broccoli, cabbage, cucumbers, squash, yams, tomatoes, eggplant, peppers, soy products, berries
Genistein	In test tubes, blocks angiogenesis, growth of new blood vessels, essential for some tumors to grow and spread, and deter proliferation of cancer cells	Found in urine of people with diets rich in soybeans and, to a lesser extent, cabbage-family vegetables

Sources: Dr. Christopher W.W. Beecher; *Eating Well Magazine;*
From: *The New York Times*, April 13, 1993

Component	Possible disease-fighting properties	Food sources
Fiber	Dilutes carcinogenic compounds in colon and speeds them through digestive system; discourages growth of harmful bacteria while bolstering healthful ones; may encourage production of healthier form of estrogen	Whole grains and many vegetables
Indoles	Induce protective enzymes	Cabbage, brussels sprouts, kale
Isothiocyanates	Induce protective enzymes	Mustard, horseradish, radishes
Limonoids	Induce protective enzymes	Citrus fruits
Linolenic acid	Regulates prostaglandin production	Many leafy vegetables and seeds, especially flaxseed
Lycopene	Antioxidant	Tomatoes, red grapefruit
Monoterpenes	Some antioxidant properties; inhibit cholesterol production in tumors; aid protective enzyme activity	Parsley, carrots, broccoli, cabbage, cucumbers, squash, yams, tomatoes, eggplant, peppers, mint, basil, citrus fruits
Phenolic acids (tannins)	Some antioxidant properties; inhibit formation of nitrosamine, a carcinogen, and affect enzyme activity	Parsley, carrots, broccoli, cabbage, tomatoes, eggplant, peppers, citrus fruits, whole grains, berries
Plant sterols, (Vitamin D precursors)	Differentiation agents	Broccoli, cabbage, cucumbers, squash, yams, tomatoes, eggplant, peppers, soy products, whole grains
Vitamin C	Antioxidant; inhibits creation of nitrosamine, a potentially dangerous carcinogen in the stomach	Citrus fruits, tomatoes, green leafy vegetables, potatoes
Vitamin E	Antioxidant	Wheat germ, oatmeal, peanuts, nuts, brown rice

Chapter Eight

Stopping the Wasteland

If we can take care of the land,
the land will take care of us.

Dick Thompson, Iowa farmer

Farming in concert with natural cycles, in ways that do not impoverish the soil and consume finite natural resources, is to farm sustainably. This is still within our reach. It is a vision that must become a reality if we want to protect and restore the natural beauty and diversity of this planet.

Human beings are creating wastelands on soil and sea. Earth has lost three billion acres of fertile soil since its inception—an area the size of China and India combined—according to the 1992 study, "Toward Sustainable Development."[1] The primary causes for soil loss are overgrazing (35 percent), deforestation, and other nonsustainable agricultural practices.

An awareness of the rhythms of nature and of natural cycles was integral to the religious and cultural traditions and agricultural practices of many preindustrial civilizations. To be connected with the earth connects us to divinity, with all that is sacred on this planet. However, industrial agriculture believes that reverence and humility toward the earth has no place in the modern world. Yet, reverence, humility, compassion, and empathy, as well as intuitive and objective knowledge, are the cornerstones of ecological farming. These values were the basis for the sustainable agriculture of human societies for millennia. These societies were successful when they sought to optimize, rather than maximize, the productivity of the land without incurring imbalance.

As an incentive for sustainable agriculture, the governments of Denmark, Finland, Austria, Norway, Sweden, Germany, and some cantons in Switzerland subsidize farmers who convert to organic farming or other sustainable farming systems that include soil and water conservation. This approach will be more economical in the long term rather than set-aside government programs designed to control over-production in conventional agriculture.

As factories and cities begin to recycle materials such as paper, glass, plastic and metal, organic sustainable farming systems begin to focus on the urgent need to restore natural agricultural cycles. One important step in restoration is to break up livestock and poultry factories and feedlots and disperse domestic animals more evenly to thrive in farming systems that are linked more closely with the dynamic cycles of ecological rather than industrial farming. The vision of dairy cows grazing in Wisconsin dales, of free-ranging hogs in harvested fields, rotational pastures, and oak and mixed evergreen woodlots, is both a romantic vision and in practical alignment with the cycles of ecological farming.

Organic Agriculture

The vernacular definition of organic agriculture means relating to, produced with, or based on the use of organics as fertilizers without employment of chemically formulated fertilizers or pesticides. Organic farming involves a number of integrated practices and components "constituting a whole whose parts are mutually dependent or intrinsically related." It is in part based on the use of organics to maintain soil quality and productivity. Organic farming has several systems and philosophies; however, theories and practices change, so the meanings of words inevitably change and the concept of organic farming continues to evolve.

The organic agriculture movement has established production standards for private certification by national and international organizations of organic farmers, such as the International Federation of Organic Farm Movements. Farmers pay a premium to have their food products examined and certified as organic. The U.S. federal government now wants to establish organic standards, which could potentially undermine present organic certification standards. If federal standards, under the Organic Food Production Act of 1990, do not satisfy cardinal bioethical criteria, then organic farmers currently certified by private organic certifiers (whose standards do address these bioethical criteria) will have no market advantage over other farmers who can claim to be organic under the lower standards set by the United States Department of Agriculture.

Bioethical Principles

1. *Ahimsa.* (avoidance of harm or injury). Organic farming seeks to minimize harm to agricultural and natural ecosystems, to wildlife, soil microorganisms, beneficial insects, and birds.

2. *Biodiversity.* Organic farming protects and even enhances biodiversity of both domestic and non-domestic animals and plants.

3. *Transgenerational equity.* This secures, and enhances the environmental quality and the productivity of the land for future generations.

4. *Enhance the life and beauty of the land.* The principle of symbiotic enhancement is a criterion that many organic, ecological farming systems exemplify. The antithesis of this is industrial farming systems that now blight much of what was, a generation or two ago, called the countryside.

For example, a dairy farmer with four thousand dairy cows in feedlots might be able to label his dairy produce as organic under federal standards, but could never qualify under current private certification programs. Skilled and dedicated organic farmers, and conscientious consumers could be losers if the U.S. Department of Agriculture sets standards below those established already by third-party certifiers; and if independent organic certifiers' verifying trademarks and seals are no longer permitted by the government.

One long-standing principle of organic agriculture is *balance*. This concept implies the maintenance of balance between inputs, productivity, and the agri-ecological resource base. This principle, loosely termed "sustainability," bears the following: All basic inputs—primarily from local resources—are natural and organic. All outputs or products are bioregionally appropriate in maximizing productivity and profitability without depleting the resource base beyond its capacity to regenerate naturally or for appropriate human intervention to restore it. This restoration may include the use of specifically approved synthetics. Depending on the bioregion, farm animals play an integral role in helping maintain balance and optimal biodiversity. Organic farming means:

♦ **The use of natural products, byproducts, and processes;**

♦ **The use of appropriate synthetic products, byproducts, and processes;**

♦ **The design and adoption of cost-efficient crop, livestock, and poultry production practices.**

These organic farming principles seek to mimic natural ecosystems in energy flow, conservation, and sustainable productivity.

A major study of biodynamic organic farming practices in New Zealand dispels the fear that organic farming is not financially viable. The results showed: "The physical, biological, and chemical soil properties and economic profitability of adjacent, commercial biodynamic and conventional farms (sixteen total) in New Zealand were compared. The biodynamic farms in the study had better soil quality than the neighboring conventional farms and were just as financially viable on a per hectare basis."[2] It is interesting to note that biodynamically farmed soil averaged 175 earthworms per square meter compared with 21 worms per square meter from conventionally farmed soils. Earthworms are important because they make and aerate soil and enhance moisture retention.

The same New Zealand study revealed that several farmers switched to more sustainable practices because of their concern about chemicals in the food chain. The cost of such inputs—animal health and welfare and groundwater pollution from agrichemicals and animal wastes from factory farms—also concerned them.

The transformation of our dysfunctional, unhealthy agricultural system into one that links closely with natural cycles and principles of organic systems and holistic resource management will take time. Governments must help farmers financially to get off the agrichemical treadmill by phasing out subsidies to those who use pesticides and other agrichemicals and who do not adopt sustainable ecological farming methods. For instance, shifting to a grass-fed livestock production system in the United States would free up three hundred million tons of grain per year for export,[3] enough to feed four hundred million people.[4] (In turn, the consequences of exporting grain for food dependency would have to be weighed carefully against spending U.S. dollars to provide aid and development programs to countries fostering sustainable agriculture and self-reliance.)

Certainly, the United States needs to raise more grass to sustain forage-fed livestock instead of using millions of Midwest acres of former prairie, woodlands, and wetlands to raise corn and soybeans for feeding livestock at home and abroad. Fortunately, many farmers and agricultural scientists are changing feeding practices, relying more on forages—like alfalfa and highly nutritious grasses—and crop rotations to help reduce soil erosion and to enrich and sanitize the soil.

Many farmers are discovering the financial benefits of sustainable farming. For example, Joel Salatin raises broiler chickens on a pasture in Virginia.[5] This practice cut feed costs by 30 percent.[6] Iowa State University animal scientist, Mark Honeyman, Ph.D. shows how to replace more than 90 percent of sow feed and 10 percent to 20 percent of growing-finishing feeds for pigs with forage or byproduct feeds.[7, 8] Animal scientist, Bill Liebhardt, Ph.D.,[9] of the University of California demonstrates that when dairy farms switched from confinement feeding to intensive rotational grazing, they had feed-cost savings of up to 36 percent.[10]

Humane Sustainable Agriculture

There are growing numbers of farmers and ranchers who care and support the humane movement. A revolution is gaining momentum internationally to make agriculture more ecologically sound, and environmentally and consumer friendly.

The essence of progress is to apply science and ethics in a sane, logical way. We must develop and adopt agricultural practices and invest in industries that cause the least harm and create the greatest good for the entire world community. In the application of science, we cannot sacrifice the welfare of the environment or of rural communities for the short-term good of the economy. If we do, then society will suffer greatly, if not this generation, then the next. Likewise, we cannot sacrifice the well-being of farm animals or of the soil in the name of productivity and technological innovation.

A humane sustainable agriculture is farming with compassion and consideration for land and animals. Environmentally sound land management produces adequate amounts of safe, wholesome food in a way that is ecologically and economically viable, equitable, and humane. Humane sustainable agriculture offers society a way by which we can eat with conscience—a way to support compassionate care of the environment and animals.

The major criteria for bioethical evaluation demonstrate the interconnectedness of these interdependent elements, which all converge on economics or full-cost accounting. These bioethical criteria include:

♦ **Safety and effectiveness;**

♦ **Social justice, equity, and farm animal well-being;**

♦ **Environmental impact, including harm to wildlife, loss of ecosystems and biodiversity;**

♦ **Socio-economic and cultural impact, especially harm to established sustainable practices and communities;**

♦ **Accord with established organic and other humane sustainable agriculture practices, standards and production claims.**

As mentioned, at the core of the principle of bioethics is the compassionate concept of *ahimsa*, which means nonharmful and nonviolent action. *Ahimsa* avoids harm to other living beings, human and nonhuman, plant and animal, wild and domesticated, either directly, or indirectly by damaging the environment. (See "Bioethical Principles" page 145.) Mahatma Gandhi, one of the great proponents of the doctrine of *ahimsa*, clarified this ideal:

> Strictly speaking, no activity or industry is possible without a certain amount of violence, no matter how little. Even the very process of living is impossible without a certain amount of violence. What we have to do is to minimize it to the greatest extent possible. Indeed the very word non-violence, a negative word, means that it is an effort to abandon the violence that is inevitable in life. Therefore, whoever believes in *Ahimsa* will engage themselves in occupations that involve the least possible violence.[11]

'Sustainable' Farms are Competitive

In a survey of 453 Minnesota farmers, the Northwest Area Foundation found that "sustainable" farmers — those who rely less on chemicals and give more attention to crop rotation, erosion control, and soil regeneration — tend to have smaller farms and substantially lower gross incomes than their more conventional counterparts. Sustainable farmers also claim less in government subsidies. But once the bills are paid, the net incomes from the two types of farms are similar. The incomes reported below are for 1989.

Farm Size

Sustainable farms - 361 acres
Conventional farms - 623 acres

Median Government Subsidy

Sustainable farms - $3,597
Conventional farms - $9,214

Median Gross Income

Sustainable farms - $ 58,750
Conventional farms - $105,999

Median Net Income

Sustainable farms - $17,451
Conventional farms - $22,836

Source: Northwest Area Foundation and the University of Minnesota

In order to avoid the costs and consequences of intensive, animal-based industrial agriculture, first and foremost we need to have a soil-based agriculture. One that uses various crops, forages, and animal species sustainably within the limits of available renewable local natural resources.

Sustainable farmers tend to have smaller farms and substantially lower gross incomes than their more conventional counterparts according to a report by the Northwest Area Foundation (NAF).[12] These are the farmers who rely less on chemicals and give more attention to crop rotation, erosion control, and soil regeneration. Livestock operations are more prevalent on sustainable farms and are less likely to use hormones and/or antibiotics than do conventional farms. Sustainable farmers also claim less in government subsidies. Once they pay their bills, the net incomes from the two types of farms are similar.

The conclusion of the NAF report is that a gradual switch to more sustainable farming practices may prove less financially threatening to conventional farmers than many fear. The Northwest Area Foundation will next evaluate what such a switch might do to agriculture production and consumer food prices. It is likely that farmers going through the transition from conventional to more sustainable agriculture will experience some financial losses during the first two to four years. During this transitional time, some financial support and subsidies from enlightened governments are in order.

In the long term, this would reap significant benefits to society since, as this study has shown, sustainable farms are actually less dependent on government subsidies than conventional farms because they are producing and marketing a greater diversity of crops for local consumption. As it stands now, commodity crops for multinational corporations to sell to their contracted livestock producers or to export are heavily subsidized.

One way to deal with the chronic problem of subsidy-stimulated overproduction is for the government to help provide the market incentives for farmers to develop new crops, like hemp for paper and textiles, varieties of soybeans for making tofu rather than for livestock feed, and nutritious cereals like quinoa, spelt, and keff.

Farm Animals in Sustainable Agriculture

Agriculture is a biological system, and works best with an integrated approach. Alternative agriculture ecologists are reaffirming the many benefits of raising different animal species together. The diversity, productivity, and nutritive value of rangeland plants increase when different species, for example, sheep, goats, and cattle, graze in a particular cycle. Mixed-species grazing also controls some parasites and certain diseases. Chickens consume disease-spreading flies, maggots, and ticks foraged from livestock manure along with a variety of nutritious seeds in the yards and night corrals. In turn, the chickens fatten and lay eggs productively. Overgrazing of key plant varieties is less likely when several species that do not eat the same plants are put together.

Another benefit of "mixed grazing" is being investigated with renewed interest since preliminary studies show that a cow can be a sheep's best friend. United States Department of Agriculture field researchers in New Mexico have confirmed that putting sheep and cattle together cut coyote-caused losses to zero. According to the USDA, sheep losses cost ranchers nearly $5 million each year. Researchers confined young sheep and cattle together in corrals to "bond" before turning them out on the range. On the range, the cattle intimidated coyotes and deterred them from attacking sheep. Scientists are seeking to identify individual sheep that form the strongest bonds with cattle, and then hope to breed the trait into other animals.

Goats, sheep, and cattle can also help control weeds on plantations. Chickens, ducks, and geese are a safer and more productive alternative to herbicides and pesticides in fields, gardens, and orchards for controlling weeds and insects. Farm animals can also help control diseases. For example, chickens eat ticks that often infect livestock and humans with various diseases. Pigs help clean up crop residues, reduce plant pathogens, and help control weeds by rooting the soil. The excrement of these creatures also helps enrich the soil.

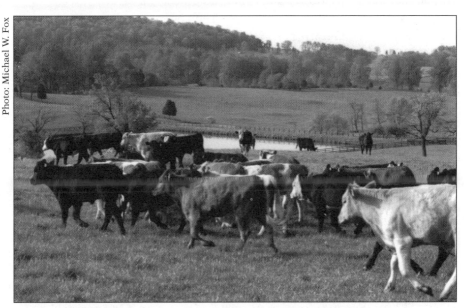

With sustainable agriculture, farm animals can help maintain good rangeland.

Agricultural entomologist Stuart Gage at Michigan State University is one scientist now demonstrating the value of geese in controlling weeds and insect pests in orchards.[13] Gage has shown that geese introduced into the orchard can replace pesticides and herbicides. Herbicide use can also be reduced by using young geese to control weeds in certain crops such as strawberries.[14] Muscovy ducks can control house flies. The house fly spreads disease and costs farmers in the United States alone an estimated $60 million a year.[15]

Farm animals can also help in maintaining healthy rangelands and permanent pastures that help collect and purify the rains and feed the rivers from their vast watershed. These rangelands help revitalize the atmosphere by absorbing such greenhouse gases as carbon dioxide and methane.

While many vegetarian-animal rights activists advocate the abolition of all animal agriculture, the elimination of farm animals from crop-integrated, and other more sustainable farming systems, is ecologically naive. Farm animals are important plant nutrient recyclers. In the absence of their beneficial manure and grazing activities, a macrocycle of ecological farming is difficult to achieve.

When farmers and horticulturists become organic, or reduce the use of chemicals by adopting an integrated pest management control program, they turn to nature for help. They encourage beneficial birds and insects to help control crop pests. In order to do so, they plant suitable cover and particular wild plants and create microhabitats that attract these creatures. These animals become the organic farmers' employees and allies. The better care they receive, the better the ecology of the farming system functions.

By working with nature, the farmer makes a quantum leap in farming without harm and experiences a radical change in attitude. The old adversarial attitude toward nature and wildlife becomes one of increasing cooperation and respect. This new knowledge base leads to a mutually enhanced symbiosis with other life forms and with the forces and processes of nature. The final product—food for humans—is not seen as some profitable commodity but as the fruit of a more meaningful way of life that is profitable, and not at nature's expense.

The Seven Principles of Humane Organic Sustainable Agriculture

1. Humane organic sustainable agriculture (HOSA) entails the production of crops and domestic animal protein and fiber on the economically prudent basis of an ecologically sound animal husbandry. Such husbandry aims to enhance or at least protect the natural biodiversity of indigenous wild plant and animal species, and does not result in environmental degradation and pollution.

2. HOSA is socially just, respecting human rights and interests, especially those of indigenous peoples and native, peasant, and family-farm cultures and traditions. The preservation of cultural diversity has inherent value in the same way as the preservation and enhancement of biodiversity.

3. HOSA recognizes the connections between consumer health and farm animal health and well-being. It respects the right of consumers of animal protein to wholesome and healthful produce. This produce comes from animals whose basic physiological, behavioral and social needs—which are integral to their overall health and well-being—are fully satisfied by the humane methods of husbandry. This minimizes the use of veterinary drugs to maintain animal health and productivity. Farmers adopt humane animal husbandry practices that in turn lowers consumer health risks. Furthermore, HOSA maximizes animals' health and overall well-being rather than sacrificing them to maximize productivity. Optimal productivity is linked with maximal animal welfare. This in turn links the optimal carrying capacity of the environment with availability of renewable natural resources.

4. HOSA is bioregionally appropriate, if not autonomous, linking livestock and poultry production with ecologically sound, organic or minimally chemical-dependent crop and forage production systems, and environmentally sound rangeland management, as the case may be.

5. HOSA does not engage in the import or export of any agricultural commodities, especially meat, wool, hides and animal foodstuffs, that are produced at the expense of natural biodiversity and nonrenewable resources. HOSA does not undermine the rights and interests of indigenous peoples and local farmers who practice ecologically sustainable, economically viable and socially just agriculture.

6. I base HOSA philosophically upon the aphorism that we do not inherit the land, we borrow it from our children, and that it is ours only in sacred trust. This means, therefore, that HOSA entails respect and reverence for all life, its philosophy being Creation—or Earth-centered. It therefore embraces concern for the rights and interests of people, animals and the environment. By so doing, it reconciles conflicting claims and concerns with the absolute rights of all life to a whole and healthy environment and to equal and fair consideration.

7. HOSA provides the foundation for a community of hope and of a planetary democracy, whereby world peace, justice, and the integrity of creation may be better assured.

Chapter Nine

Change of Conscience:
Actions and Solutions

*The significant problems of the world
cannot be solved at the same level of consciousness
at which they were created.*

Albert Einstein

The problems that our now dysfunctional industrial agriculture has created are complex, but the consumer public is not helpless. Much can be done to put agriculture back on an ecologically sound basis and to put farm animals back into green pastures. We can make change simply by making different purchasing decisions.

If we do not start to change our dietary habits, the agricultural problems in both developed and less-developed countries will continue to multiply. We cannot expect governments to act on our behalf if we refuse to do anything for ourselves. Now is the time to act.

As citizen-consumers, we can do much to stop the wasteland from spreading. At this time there are two kinds of agriculture in America; the ecological small family farms, and the larger industrial farms that are integrated with agribusiness corporations. Big business is pushing the more environmentally and consumer-friendly farming systems out of business. As consumers we can help stop this in many ways. One of the most immediate actions consumers can take is to get involved to ensure that labeling is required on all food products. This is the only way you will truly know what you are eating. Labeling can include all ingredients as well as all farm animal products stating the region or country of origin, and describe the raising methods (free-ranging, humanely grown) and whether or not antibiotics, chemicals, or pesticides were used. By labeling organic and humanely grown food, the necessary market niche for farmers and ranchers who share the vision of greener pastures will be secure.

The democratic rights of consumers to be informed must prevail. See the listed resources at the back of this book for more information and involvement. Below are suggestions for immediate consumer action. You decide where to begin, and take the next step.

Initiatives for Concerned and Conscientious Consumers

♦ Get involved in an organization that works for the welfare of animals on a local as well as a national level. There are some effective and committed groups of people nationally and internationally who are making a difference in animal welfare. As an example, nonprofit organizations such as the Humane Farming Association and Farm Sanctuary, have a "No Downer Campaign," which is pushing for national legislation to ban "downed" animal cruelties by eliminating the economic incentive for the meat industry to deal in "downers." *The Downed Animal Protection Act* (H.R. 453) prohibits the sale of downed animals at livestock markets through the United States. See *Resources* for organizations involved in animal welfare.

♦ Get your hands dirty by planting trees in your neighborhood or community, or getting involved on a global level by supporting environmental groups such as Rainforest Action Network and Earth Island Institute, which are working to protect the rainforests that are still left. Trees are the lungs of the earth and billions of acres have been cleared worldwide to open up land for grazing cattle. Trees, along with sea plankton, help reduce global warming by absorbing carbon dioxide, and provide the oxygen all breathing creatures need.

♦ Writing letters to government agencies and state representatives in Congress can influence public policy and legislation. First, you need to have some background information on the issues that concern you, and the various organizations and their publications listed in the Resources at the end of this book will be invaluable in this regard. They need your support as a concerned citizen and consumer. Many of their regular publications provide details on critical issues and pending legislation that need public support, and to whom your valuable letters should be sent.

♦ Writing letters and editorials for your local newspaper can also stir up the uninformed and bring critical food, animal, and farming issues before the public. Agencies such as the federal Food and Drug Administration and the United States Department of Agriculture do respond to letters from the public, and your state legislators and congressional representatives will take note. Not all politicians are in the pockets of the agribusiness food industry. They know that it is your vote that keeps them in office. You can demand public hearings for local issues such as where the food in school lunch programs comes from or on a new hog factory that is being built in your county.

♦ If there is a university in your county that has an agriculture department, find out what they are doing and challenge those programs and research activities that do not benefit in-state family farms, rural communities, and local concerns. Many are doing contract research for multinational food and drug corporations often partly funded by state tax dollars. They need to have their priorities and mission put on the right track.

♦ If there is a community college, or elementary and high schools in your area, find out what they are teaching in home economics and nutrition courses and what materials from the meat and dairy industries are being used. With a little encouragement, they may invite courses in vegetarian cooking or eating with conscience. Perhaps the school would be interested in working with local organic farmers to buy food for the school's needs.

♦ Survey your local restaurants and hotels and find out which offer one or more vegetarian entrées, and let your local newspaper know. Make up lists of supermarkets and smaller food stores that provide organic foods, eggs from free-range, uncaged hens, produce from local and in-state farms, and other goods from community coops. Share with friends and become an "eating with conscience" community networker.

♦ Keep good food from being wasted. Ask supermarkets, restaurants, and caterers where unsold perishables go. In many communities, the local shelters for the homeless, soup kitchens, and food banks can make good use of such products.

♦ When you eat out and you enjoyed a meatless meal, ask to see the chef and give your praise. Chefs like to please their clients, and words of praise may encourage the chef to try more vegan and vegetarian recipes and to join the revolutionary Chefs' Collaborative 2000. (See "Chefs Join the Revolution" later in this chapter.) Be venturesome and explore new recipes based on tofu and various beans, and visit local ethnic restaurants to educate your palate and discover new meatless dishes.

♦ Have friends over for a vegetarian or vegan dinner. Hold a school picnic that is all vegetarian (with real fruit drinks!). Have a caterer make a vegetarian or vegan buffet for a party at home or at the office. When you fly, order a vegan or vegetarian meal in advance. If you are going to a convention with a meal check-off or a scheduled banquet, ask the organizers to put you down for "vegetarian." In such instances I have often found my vegetarian meal to be the envy of others at my table who got stuck with the usual rubber chicken, iceberg lettuce, and vanilla swirl ice cream.

♦ If you have children at school or college who embrace eating with conscience, help them get the administration to provide meatless meals and a vegetarian/vegan choice for all students and faculty.

♦ Grow some of your own food. Or use a community garden commons or even a vacant lot as many people are now doing in urban areas.

♦ As a conscientious consumer, recycle your garbage, and learn how to compost some of the garbage for your garden or community plot. In some neighborhoods, farmers, horticulturists, and market gardeners will pick up compostable garbage.

♦ Some socially responsible individuals have brought farmers and small-scale fruit and vegetable producers, local bakers and other foodmakers into town, and designated Saturday as the food-market day in a corner of the shopping mall parking lot, a school playground, public park, or town square. These farmers' and food markets give new life to communities and make a fun outing for all.

♦ Since local farmers in most parts of the United States do not produce food throughout the year, you may want to explore old and new ways of seeing yourself and your family through the lean months by freezing, pickling, canning, bottling, and drying various local produce. Some foods, depending on the variety, like onions, potatoes, yams, apples, pears, and squashes will stay fresh if they are stored in a cool, dry place like our grandparents' root cellars. Do not forget you can have fresh greens every day throughout the winter in the form of sprouted wheat, cress, alfalfa, and a host of other nutritious seeds that are tasty chopped up. You can grow herbs indoors in the winter and even mushrooms.

♦ Avoid the temptation of eating fruits and vegetables out of season that have been imported, often without any label as to country of origin, and often from countries where there are virtually no pesticide regulations. Many agrichemicals banned in this country (but manufactured here nonetheless) are on and in the produce you buy. Small amounts may not harm you, but think of the harm to farmworkers and wildlife.

♦ Avoid purchasing processed foods, junk-food snacks and "meals" in a box or freezer pack. The more meals that you prepare at home from basic ingredients (ideally organic), the more you will be breaking up the market monopoly of food giants and asserting your independence by eating with conscience. (Less paper and plastic packaging is generated as well.)

♦ Pay attention to urban sprawl in your community or city. The American Farmland Trust estimates that we are losing about one million acres of good farm land every year because of suburban spread—*which is about two acres every minute!* Citizens can stop this by insisting on stricter zoning laws or protecting the ones that are already in place. Citizens can also lobby for conservation-easement covenants to help protect farmland and open spaces from real estate speculators and developers. You might be amazed at how much difference a handful of activists can make. There are many inspiring stories of individuals and neighborhood groups who tackled the "Goliaths" of urban sprawl and won!

The Ten Commandments of Humane Organic Sustainable Agriculture:

A Pledge for Farmers, Ranchers, and Consumers

1. Make a covenant to transform conventional industrialized agriculture into a profitable and equitable system of food and fiber production that is humane and ecologically sound.

2. Practice and support agricultural methods that are good for all: for farmers, ranchers, the land, animals, and consumers.

3. Support local farms and farmers' markets in the community or region that offer produce from organic and other alternative sustainable methods of food production.

4. If you are not a vegetarian, purchase no animal produce from factory farms where veal calves, pigs, and poultry are raised in complete confinement, never having access to the outdoors, and factory feedlots where thousands of cows and beef cattle are kept in dirt lots often without shade or shelter.

5. Support state and federal legislation and civil initiatives to encourage the adoption of humane organic sustainable agriculture (HOSA) and discourage the proliferation of factory farming.

6. Stay informed and involved by joining one or more of the organizations listed in the Resources section of this book.

7. Commit to informing others about why supporting HOSA is good for you and good for all. Be part of the alliance between urban consumers and rural producers to farm without harm and eat with conscience.

8. Reach out and encourage local institutions—schools, hospitals, church groups—to engage in community supported agriculture.

9. Appeal to grocery stores and restaurants to provide certified organic foods, more humane animal products, such as eggs from uncaged hens, free-range pork and beef, and rBGH-hormone free dairy products.

10. Refine the food you eat by purchasing only organic, humanely and sustainably obtained meat, eggs, and dairy products. Reduce your consumption of all high fat, low fiber products. Replace them with whole grains, beans, vegetables, and fruits—organic whenever possible.

Chefs Join the Revolution

Chefs are now uniting in opposition against agribusiness and genetically engineered foods. They are beginning to realize their role in helping to facilitate industrial agriculture's transition to a more organic, ecological, humane, and equitable system. One group, Chefs' Collaborative 2000, has drafted a charter to promote the growing, cooking, and eating of food. They promote eight principles for cooking in ways that will sustain the natural resources of the planet and the health of its human inhabitants. The Statement of Principles are:

1. Food is fundamental to life. It nourishes us in body and soul, and the sharing of food immeasurably enriches our sense of community;

2. Good, safe, wholesome food is a basic human right;

3. Society has the obligation to make good, pure food affordable and accessible to all;

4. Good food begins with unpolluted air, land, and water, environmentally sustainable farming and fishing, and humane animal husbandry;

5. Sound food choices emphasize locally grown, seasonally fresh and whole or minimally processed ingredients;

6. Cultural and biological diversity is essential for the health of the planet and its inhabitants. Preserving and revitalizing sustainable food and agricultural traditions strengthen that diversity;

7. The healthy traditional diets of many cultures offer abundant evidence that fruits, vegetables, beans, breads, and grains are the foundation of good diets;

8. As part of their education, our children deserve to be taught basic cooking skills and to learn the impact of their food choices on themselves, on their culture, and on their environment.[1]

Consumer Beware: Products from Animal Suffering

To be what I call a discriminating consumer takes vigilance. If you want to avoid eggs and dairy products that are not organic and from animals that are not kept humanely, read the label. You will be amazed at how many baked goods and varieties of pasta contain one or both of these animal products. Rendered parts of animals are everywhere too:

from the gelatin (from boiled hooves and horns) in cooking gelatin, marshmallows, and vitamin capsules, to the tallow or fat in our candles, floor waxes, crayons, soaps, plastic wrapping for food, camera film, face creams, lipstick, and various other cosmetics. This explains why cats like to lick plastic, photographs, and their owners' skin! Collagen, a protein extracted from bones, hides, and hooves, is in many lotions and moisturizers, and is even injected by dermatologists into people's faces to remove wrinkles.

Many subsidiary industries are dependent upon these livestock byproducts, so the very thought of people reducing or eliminating all animal products from their plates, clothes closets, and bathroom cabinets is threatening. Consumers can do fine without any animal products. But livestock-dependent industries cannot.

Pets and Pet Food

I have been outraged by another kind of factory farming that has proliferated in the Midwest, especially over the past twenty years. These are the notorious purebred dog breeding factories supplying pet stores around the world. The American Kennel Club allows pups from these factories to be registered and licensed by U.S. Department of Agriculture inspectors who should instead close down most of these "puppy mill" factories. They are a national disgrace. Parent dogs—the "breeding stock" —often spend their entire lives in long, narrow wire cages elevated a few feet above their excrement. Their offspring are often riddled with diseases and genetic defects. So consumer beware and never buy that puppy in the window that came from a breeding factory. Picket the pet shop and put it out of business!

The pet food industry is a major component of the agribusiness livestock feed and food industrial complex. The American pet food industry is a $9.2 billion a year business. It is so influential that selected employees teach nutrition courses at some veterinary colleges. Students are told that table scraps and human food are "bad" for dogs and cats. Veterinary students are not taught about pet carcasses, roadkill, condemned parts of livestock, and the inedible byproducts of the human food and beverage industries used as ingredients in pet food.

Discriminating consumers who have cats and dogs should carefully read the labels on commercial pet food and avoid all products that include any artificial preservatives like ethoxyquin and propylene glycol, or products that include meat "meal" (roadkill, dogs and cats, and discarded parts of farm animals), chicken "meal" (that may include ground-up heads, feathers, and feet), and tallow (the fat of discarded and chemically contaminated animals).

Gourmet Products to Avoid

The best that the discriminating consumer can do to avoid animal products is to read the label and if in doubt, do not buy it. In the realm of cuisine, the gourmet is regarded as a discriminating consumer. However, I question the gourmet who relishes goose liver paté from geese force-fed until their livers almost burst with fat; caviar from sturgeon fish being driven to extinction by people illegally obtaining and selling the eggs; frogs' legs prepared in most cases by simply cutting their legs in half while they are fully conscious; escargot dishes created by cooking the snails alive, and live lobsters that are boiled alive. Other gourmet meat dishes gaining in popularity are rabbit raised while crammed into wire cages; venison (from deer), and pheasant, quail, and ostrich meat obtained from wild creatures kept in small enclosures. Though they may be unusual, these animals are from factory farm systems, along with turtles and even alligators.

There are other animal products that we don't eat, but you may nonetheless want to avoid purchasing because of their owners' inhumane practices. Merino wool products are off my list. This fine wool comes from sheep packed in huge confinement sheds. The sheep never get outdoors to graze or play. I have not purchased any woolen item for over a decade. My wool winter coat was a secondhand gift. I still wear a forty-year-old tweed jacket from free-roaming Scottish moorland, Blackface sheep. This is the same coat that I wore as a veterinary student. I avoid all leather products—jackets, belts, shoes, items with fur, lizard, ostrich, or kangaroo skin trim. Canvas, hemp, and new synthetic leather substitutes (unfortunately not quickly degradable) are on my more acceptable list. Buying secondhand leather products so as to recycle them and not purchasing new leather items is another alternative. The manufacture of leather products entails the use of toxic tanning chemicals, and dyes, which cause extensive pollution of rivers and water supplies in countless less developed countries. These leather products we purchase so cheaply in America, in addition to other items such as Armani's Merino wool turtlenecks, Nike's kangaroo skin-trimmed sneakers, and Nieman Marcus ostrich skin wallets embellished with rattlesnake skin—come from animals whose fate seems to concern so few.

Other animal products produced at the cost of much suffering include the factory-scale production of silk from silk worms who are boiled alive; of duck and goose down from live birds plucked raw and confined their entire life indoors; perfume musk from the anal glands of African civet cats who are kept in small cages, often in filth and half-starved in countries such as Ethiopia; and of all the foxes, mink, chinchillas, and other wild creatures raised in small cages on factory ranches until they are killed to make fur coats. I have been sickened by the sight of mink and foxes spinning and pacing neurotically in the tiny cages they are confined to on factory fur farms. So as not to damage their pelts, they are often killed with an electrified rod shoved into their rectums. For all of the above-mentioned products there are many alternatives.

Many of these animals are fed the byproducts of the livestock and fishing industries. It is no surprise that the fur industry is afraid of the animal rights and vegetarian movements. These two movements are gaining considerable public support and are uniting their concerns with other movements such as labor, consumer nutrition, food safety, organic agriculture, and world hunger.

Perhaps some readers and critics will feel that I am going too far in delineating "politically correct" consumer choices. I abhor this notion of political correctness since it denotes a fad or trend that can change overnight with the political climate. Eating with conscience and being a discriminating consumer challenge us to maintain our ethical consistency and the bioethics of compassion and nonviolence, which are life-long work.

Community Supported Agriculture

Community Supported Agriculture (CSA) is a grassroots revolution that is making some deep roots in many parts of the United States. It works in the following manner. Several families contract with a farmer, or a cooperative network of farms, that provides them with fresh, often organic, foods for a good part of the year. Sometimes the farmer provides various recipes, baked goods, and arranges farm visits for contracting families and schools. Each household pays the farmer or farmers' cooperative a set fee in advance. This gives the farmer the necessary financial security if there's some catastrophic crop loss. Catastrophes are rare, since most CSA farms raise a variety of crops and will often make up any deficiencies in their weekly deliveries to clients by taking produce from neighbor farmers.

CSA eliminates the incredible public costs of price supports and subsidies, and there is no need for the government to buy up surplus produce to stabilize prices. Families just eat a few more potatoes or beets for a few weeks.

CSA promotes cooperation rather than competition between farmers and is most effective in forging a strong alliance between urban (and suburban) consumers and rural producers. The households who eat the CSA produce live close to where the food grows. Eating locally grown food helps cut down transportation and road maintenance costs and pollution.

Conventional agribusiness produce travels an average of twelve hundred miles before finishing up on the plate. Spoilage occurs in long-distance transportation and in produce remaining unsold in the supermarket. With direct producer-to-consumer marketing, we can save an average 25 percent of every harvest from spoilage. In conventional agriculture, we must estimate another 25 percent loss of produce that gets left in the fields because it does not meet market standards of uniformity. The CSA market does not reject bent carrots, undersize apples and potatoes, and squash and tomatoes with a few blemishes. When we total the harvest savings of CSA, it requires half the land use that conventional agriculture uses, which means more acres for nature and wildlife.

* * *

We can farm without harm, eat with conscience, heal the oceans, regenerate our land, and recover our humanity. We will know we are on the right path again when agrichemicals are rarely needed and used, when livestock factories are gone, and when food—its production and marketing—regains those sacramental elements of stewardship, communion, and thanksgiving.

Now is the time for action. We can all make a difference. As voters we can support legislation and public policy that encourage farmers to adopt humane, ecological, and healthful farming practices. If we pay attention to what we eat and how it is produced, this alone will begin a revolution in food production. As consumers we can vote with our food dollars and change our eating habits for our own good and for the good of the animal kingdom, the environment, and caring farmers. Between the consumer and the farming community, there are seeds of hope to share and to spread. They are good for us, for the planet, and for generations to come.

APPENDIX

Mad Cow Disease Fact Sheet

When the plight of British cattle and risk to consumers made the news headlines, I received so many calls about the question of mad cow disease that I had the following fact sheet prepared on this issue, in collaboration with Laurel Hopwood, an environmental and consumer health advocate in Cleveland, Ohio.

What Is Mad Cow Disease, Technically Known as Bovine Spongiform Encephalopathy (BSE)?

Spongiform encephalopathies are nervous system disorders in which nerve cells of the brain die, causing the brain to assume a spongelike appearance. BSE is the term applied to this malady because it affects cows. Clinical signs in cows affected include belligerence, confusion, and poor coordination. Presently, a brain biopsy is the only way to confirm a BSE diagnosis. BSE was first recognized in 1986. The U.S. government decreed in June 1997 that dead cows and other ruminants should not be fed back to cows or other ruminants. However, they can be fed to pigs and chickens, and pig and chicken parts can be fed to ruminants.

What Causes BSE?

Scientists call the agent believed to cause BSE a "prion," an infectious protein lacking nucleic acid. Prions are thought to multiply by setting off a chain reaction that damages nearby healthy cellular proteins, converting normal proteins into abnormal ones.

Traditional methods to destroy microbes do not work on prions. Prions show resistance to normal forms of sterilization, such as common disinfectants, ultraviolet or ionizing radiation, and autoclaving. And contaminated tissue samples fixed in the preservative, Formalin, have been found to still be infectious.

How is It Transmitted to Cows?

Prions are transmissible to other species including sheep, cats, and primates. For several centuries, a form of spongiform encephalopathy called "scrapie" has been known to afflict sheep.

For the past half century, there has been a trend toward intensified production of livestock raised for consumption. To find a use for the vast tonnage of condemned and inedible remains of slaughtered animals, they are rendered down and the protein residue is fed to billions of poultry, pigs, milk cows, and beef cattle.

Some animals that are slaughtered are diseased. Since the agent that causes spongiform encephalopathy is not easily detected or destroyed, it can end up in animal feed. The brain, spinal cord, thymus, spleen, and tonsils are the parts most suspect for contamination. There is also supporting evidence that the infectious agent of BSE can be passed from an infected cow to her unborn calf.

In Britain, where mad cow disease is most prevalent, over one hundred sixty thousand cattle have been stricken with it. Infected cattle also have been found in numerous other countries including France, Italy, Germany, Switzerland, Ireland, Canada, Portugal, and Denmark.

How Are Humans Affected?

The period between infection and clinical symptoms of BSE in cattle averages four and one-half years. During this incubation period the agent can be transmitted. Infected but asymptomatic animalsmay be slaughtered and enter the human food supply.

What Is the Human Form of Spongiform Encephalopathy?

The most common form of human spongiform encephalopathy (HSE), is Creutzfeldt-Jakob Disease (CJD), 15 percent of which is of known origin (inherited or unintentionally transmitted surgically). The average age at onset of symptoms is sixty-five. However, 85 percent of HSE randomly occurs with no known cause. Clinical signs include impairment of thought, sight, and movement due to the destruction of brain cells, and a dementia resembling that of Alzheimer's disease. Muscle spasms occur, creating rigidity and jerkiness, and there is a loss of balance. Death is inevitable and swift, usually within months.

Between 1990 and 1997, the incidence of HSE in Britain has nearly doubled and continues to increase. A new form of HSE has been diagnosed in people who have had no genetic predisposition to it. Some of the afflicted people worked closely with infected cattle; some were teenagers; all ate beef. In Britain by July 1997, nineteen people had been confirmed as having this new form of HSE, the average age of onset being twenty-seven.

The new HSE differs from CJD in that there is no genetic predisposition, it has a ten-year incubation period, the microscopic appearance of the diseased nerve cells is different, and victims die within one year of exhibiting symptoms. As with cattle, the primary symptom is dementia. HSE can very easily be confused with Alzheimer's disease, which millions of people are diagnosed with each year. The cause of dementia is reportedly misdiagnosed 25 percent of the time. A postmortem microscopic examination of the brain is presently the only method available to confirm a diagnosis of HSE.

What Steps Are Being Taken?

No cases of BSE have been confirmed in the United States, and since 1989 the importation of live ruminants (cattle, sheep, etc.) and ruminant products from countries known to have BSE have been restricted. In other countries, cattle showing symptoms of BSE are killed. As of March 1996, the European Union banned the exportation of cattle, beef, and most beef byproducts from Britain. In the United States, major sheep producers claim to be voluntarily diverting sheep byproducts from cattle feed. The Food and Drug Administration (FDA) had proposed a ban on sheep tissue in cattle feed in 1994, but took no action because of strong opposition from the livestock industry. They are now proposing a mandatory ban to prohibit the use of all ruminant byproducts in cattle feed.

Is the Problem Under Control in the United States?

Some cattle imported from Britain before the 1989 ban are still here. Sheep scrapie (which has been implicated as the cause of BSE) also exists here. Despite the voluntary ban on sheep byproducts in cattle feed, FDA officials admit it is very difficult to verify compliance because there is no way to test a rendered product for sheep content. Therefore, potentially infectious animal tissue is still being fed to cattle, and infected but asymptomatic animals may still enter the human food supply.

Additionally, some three dozen marketed drugs are derived from cattle tissue and organs, and hundreds more contain bovine blood. Gelatin, derived from cattle hooves, hides, and bones is an ingredient of many foods and drugs and is used to make vitamin and pharmacapsules. The FDA is now considering formalizing a ban on the use of pharmaceutical gelatin imported from countries with BSE.

What Can I Do to Reduce My Risk of Acquiring HSE?

The best way to protect yourself is to eliminate from your diet any source of beef that may be contaminated. Intensive livestock production systems may promote BSE because animals in intensive confinement are more likely to be fed animal remains. Therefore, eliminating meat from intensive confinement or factory farms is a good start. Some organic cattle farmers in Britain believe that organophosphate pesticides, widely used on other cattle, may play a role in BSE. There have been no documented cases of BSE in cows born and raised on organic farms.

The best way of knowing what is going into your food is to know where your food comes from. Whenever possible, buy locally grown food from organic and sustainable farmers and ranchers. Let your grocers know that you want to buy local, organic produce, and animal products obtained through more humane and sustainable production methods.

References

Lawrence K. Altman. "Mad cow epidemic puts spotlight on puzzling human brain disease." *New York Times*. April 2, 1996.

Lawrence Altman. "Officials assert existing policies will safeguard beef supply." *New York Times*. March 27, 1996.

Lawrence K. Altman. "U.S. officials confident that mad cow disease of Britain has not occurred here." *Wall Street Journal*. March 27, 1996.

Lawrence K. Altman. "W.H.O. seeks barriers against cow disease." *New York Times*. April 4, 1996.

American Veterinary Medical Association. "Bovine spongiform encephalopathy (BSE) 1996 update." Issue Brief. March 27, 1996.

Sandra Blakeslee. "New understanding of how a protein runs amok." *Science*. August 16, 1994.

Marilyn Chase. "U.S. groups move to make cattle feed safe for food chain." *Wall Street Journal*. April 1, 1996.

Julian Earl. "Origin of BSE." *The Veterinary Record*. March 23, 1996.

Ian Elliott. "EU bans British beef from rest of world." *Feedstuffs*. April 1, 1996.

Ian Elliott. "Link assumed between BSE and human neurological Disease," *Feedstuffs*. March 25, 1996.

John Darnton. "British beef banned in France and Belgium." *New York Times*. March 22, 1996.

Appendix

"Link assumed between BSE and human neurological disease." *Feedstuffs*. March 25, 1996.

"British expert panel links CJD cases to BSE exposure." *Food Chemical News*. March, 25, 1996.

"British government criticized by Lancet for statements that U.K. beef is safe; new CJD strain lesions similar to scrapie." *Food Chemical News*. April 8, 1996.

"1,459 British, Irish cattle in U.S.; 42 British cats affected by BSE." *Food Chemical News*. September 13, 1993.

"USDA pledges to step up BSE surveillance in light of British experience." *Food Chemical News*. April 1, 1996.

"U.S. ruminant-to-ruminant feed ban proposal to be ready soon; voluntary ban announced by livestock and animal health groups." *Food Chemical News*. April 8, 1996.

Lacey, Richard W., *Mad Cow Disease*. Channel Islands, France: Cypsela Publications Limited. 1994.

Anita Manning. "'Mad cow' human deaths blamed on new disease strain." *USA Today*. April 5, 1996.

W.A. Marks. "Cerebral degenerations producing dementia. *"Journal of Geriatrics-Psychology-Neurology."* 1(4). Fall 1988.

Richard Marsh and William Wustenburg. "Is it safe to feed meat and bone meal?" *Hoard's Dairyman*. 1990.

Daniel Pearl. "From lipstick to marshmallows, it's got some cow in it." *Wall Street Journal*. April 3, 1996.

Mark Purdey. "Beating peril of BSE." Letter to the Editor. *Daily Express*, March 22, 1996.

Reuters, March 26, 1996 (America OnLine).

Susan Watts. "A bogeyman among the beef-eaters." *New Scientist*. February 1995.

Rick Weiss. "Link between rare human brain ailment, mysterious cow disease baffles scientists." *Washington Post*. March 26, 1996.

Robin Young. "Supplies of safe meat cannot be quickly increased." *Times*. December 9, 1995.

RESOURCES
Organizations and Publications

Acres USA
PO Box 8800
Metairie, LA 70011
504-889-2100; fax: 504-889-2777

Agriculture and Human Values Journal
Kluwer Academic Publishers
3300 AH Dordrecht
The Netherlands
31-78-6 392 393; fax: 31-78-6546474
website: www.wkap.nl

AgScene
Compassion in World Farming
Copse House, Greatham
Liss, Hampshire
England
44-730-264208

Alternative Agriculture News
Henry A. Wallace Institute for Alternative Agriculture
9200 Edmonston Road, Suite 117
Greenbelt, MD 20770
301-441-8777; fax: 301-220-0164

American Anti-Vivisection Society
Henry A. Wallace Institute for Alternative Agriculture
9200 Edmonston Road, Suite 117
Greenbelt, MD 20770
301-441-8777; fax: 301-220-0164

American Farmland, Membership Magazine of
801 Old York Road, Suite 209
Jenkintown, PA 19046-1685
800-729-2287; fax: 215-887-2088
web site: www.aavs.org

American Livestock Breeds Conservancy News
American Livestock Breeds Conservancy
Box 477
Pittsboro, NC 27312
919-542-5704; fax: 919-545-0022

Animal Activist Alert
HSUS News
The Humane Society of the United States
2100 L Street, NW
Washington, DC 20037
202-452-1100; fax: 202-778-6132

Association for Veterinarians for Animal Rights
PO Box 208
Davis, CA 95617-9903

Campaign for Sustainable Agriculture Update
PO Box 396
Pine Bush, NY 12566
914-744-8448; fax: 914-744-8477

Center for Agroecology and Sustainable Food Systems
University of California
1156 High Street
Santa Cruz, CA 95064
408-459-4140; fax: 408-459-2799

Center for Rural Affairs Newsletter
Center for Rural Affairs
PO Box 406
Walthill, NE 68067
402-846-5428; fax: 402-846-5420

Chefs' Collaborative 2000
25 First Street
Cambridge, MA 02141
617-621-3000
fax: 617-621-1230

Citizens for a Better Environment
407 S. Dearborn, Suite 1775
Chicago, IL 60605
312-939-1530; or 312-939-1984 for Public Outreach and Education;
fax: 312-939-2536

Committee for Sustainable Agriculture
406 Main Street, Suite 313
Watsonville, CA 95076
408-763-2111

Earth Island Institute
300 Broadway
Suite 28
San Francisco, CA 94133
415-788-3666
web site: www.earthisland.org

Earth Save Membership Newsletter
Earth Save International
706 Frederick
Santa Cruz, CA 95062-2205
800-362-3648; fax: 408-458-0255

Earthtrust
25 Kaneohe Bay Drive, Suite 205
Kailua, HI 96734
808-254-2866; fax: 808-254-6409
web site: www.earthtrust.org
email: whale@lava.net

Eating with Conscience Campaign
The Humane Society of the United States
2100 L Street, NW
Washington, DC 20037
301-548-7709; or 301-258-3054
fax: 301-258-3081
web site: www.hsus.org
email: ewcp@ix.netcom.com

The Ecologist
Vol. 22:4 (July-August 1992), pp. 121-216
MIT Press Journals
55 Hayward Street
Cambridge, MA 02142
617-253-2889; fax: 617-577-1545

The Envirolink Network (Internet)
4618 Henry Street
Pittsburgh, PA 15213
412-683-6400; fax: 412-683-8460
web site: www.envirolink.org

Farm Aid News and Views (monthly)
Farm Aid Update (quarterly)
PO Box 228
Champaign, IL 61824
1-800-FARM AID; fax: 617-354-6992

Farm and Food News
The Journal of the Farm and Food Society
4 Willifield Way
London NW11 7XT England
441-81-455-0634

Farm Animal Reform Movement (FARM)
Box 30654
Bethesda, MD 20824
301-530-1737; fax: 301-530-5747; 800-MEATOUT
email: FARM@gnn.com
web site: www.envirolink/arrs/farm/index.htm

Food & Water Journal
Food & Water, Inc.
RR#1, Box 68D
Walden, VT 05873
802-563-3300; fax: 802-563-3310

Friends of Animals Action Line
777 Post Road
Darien, CT 06820
203-656-1522; fax: 203-656-0267
email: foa@igc.apc.org
web site: www.friendsofanimals.com

Global Pesticide Campaigner
Pesticide Action Network
North America Regional Center
116 New Montgomery #810
San Francisco, CA 94105
415-541-9140; fax: 415-541-9253

Good Medicine Newsletter
Physicians Committee for Responsible Medicine
5100 Wisconsin Avenue, NW, Suite 404
Washington, DC 20016
202-686-2210; fax: 202-686-2216

The Green Guide for Everyday Life
Mothers and Others for a Liveable Planet
Outreach Director
40 West 20th Street
New York, NY 10011
212-242-0010, ext. 304; fax: 212-242-0545

Healthy Harvest V: A Directory of Sustainable Agriculture and Horticulture Organizations 1998
Ag Access
603 Fourth Street
Davis, CA 95616
916-756-7177; fax: 916-756-7188

Holistic Resource Management Quarterly
Center for Holistic Resource Management
1010 Tijeras, NW
Albuquerque, NM 87102
505-842-5252; fax: 505-843-7900

Humane Farming Association
76 Belvedere Street, Suite D
San Rafael, CA 94901
415-485-1495; fax: 415-485-0106

International Federation of Organic Agriculture Movement
Ecology & Farming
Okozentrum Imsbach
D-66636
Tholey-Theley , Germany
49-6853-5190; fax: 49-6853-30110

Journal of Agricultural and Environmental Ethics
Room 039, MacKinnon Building
University of Guelph
Guelph, Ontario, Canada N1G 2W1
519-824-4120, ext. 6925; fax: 519-837-9953

Journal of Soil and Water Conservation
Soil and Water Conservation Society
7515 Northeast Ankeny Road
Ankeny, IA 50021
515-289-2331; fax: 515-289-1227

The Land Report Quarterly Newsletter
The Land Institute
2440 E. Water Well Road
Salina, KS 67401
913-823-5376

The Land Stewardship Letter
Land Stewardship Project
2200 Fourth Street
White Bear Lake, MN 55110
612-653-0618

Leopold Letter
Leopold Center for Sustainable Agriculture
209 Curtiss Hall, Iowa State University
Ames, IA 50011-1050
515-294-3711; fax: 515-294-9696

National Agricultural Library
Animal Welfare Information Center
10301 Baltimore Avenue
Beltsville, MD 20705
301-504-6212; fax: 301-504-7125
email: awic@nal.usda.gov
web site: www.nal.usda.gove/awic

The Organic Report
Organic Trade Association
PO Box 1078
Greenfield, MA 01302
413-774-7511

Pigs, A Sanctuary
PO Box 629
Charlestown, WV 25414
304-725-7447; fax: 304-725-7447

Prairie Journal
Prairie Fire
550 11th Street, #200
Des Moines, IA 50309
515-274-6468

Pure Food Campaign
860 Highway 61 East
Little Marais, MN 55614
218-226-4164; fax: 218-226-4157

Rainforest Action Network
221 Pine Street, Suite 500
San Francisco, CA 94104
415-398-4404

Sanctuary News
Farm Sanctuary
PO Box 150
Watkins Glen, NY 14891
607-583-2225; 607-583-2041

Saving the Farm: A Handbook for Conserving Agricultural Land
American Farmland Trust, One Short Street
Northampton, MA 01060
800-370-4879; fax: 413-586-9332

Small-Scale Agriculture Today
US Department of Agriculture/CSREES
Room 342-A, 901 D Street, SW
Washington, DC 20250-2200
202-401-4385

State of the World Annual Report
Worldwatch Institute, 1776 Massachusetts Avenue, NW
Washington, DC 20036
202-452-1999; fax: 202-296-7365

United Poultry Concerns, Inc.
PO Box 59367
Potomac, MD   20859
301-948-2406

Viva Vegie Society
PO Box 294, Prince St. Station
New York, NY 10012
212-274-8988
email: pamela@wwonline-ny.com

Woman's International Pharmacy
57088 Monona Drive
Madison, WI   53716-3152
800-279-5708; fax: 800-279-8011
web site: www.wipws.com

World Ark
Heifer Project International
1015 S. Louisiana
Little Rock, AR 72202
501-376-6836

World Society for Sustainable Agriculture Newsletter
8554 Melrose Avenue
West Hollywood, CA 90069
213-657-7202; fax: 213-657-3884

World Society for the Protection of Animals
29 Perkins St., PO Box 190
Boston, MA 02130
617-522-7000; fax: 617-522-7077

Additional Web Site Resources

Alt Vet Med
www.altvetmed.com

Amazing Environmental Organization Web Directory
www.webdirectory.com

Animal Rights Resource Site
www.envirolink.org/arrs/homepages.html

The Animal Welfare Institute
www.animalwelfare.com

People for the Ethical Treatment of Animals
www.peta-online.org/

Vegetarian Pages
www.veg.org/veg/

World Society for the Protection of Animals
http://way.net/wspa

SELECT BIBLIOGRAPHY

W. Berry. *The Gift of Good Land*. San Francisco: North Point Press. 1981.

————. *The Unsettling of America: Culture and Agriculture*. New York: Avon. 1978.

E.A.R. Bird, G.L. Bultena, and J.C. Gardner. *Planting the Future: Developing an Agriculture that Sustains Land and Community*. Ames, IA: Iowa University Press. 1995.

J.N. Blenden, editor. *Dirt Rich, Dirt Poor. America's Food and Farm Crisis*. New York: Routledge. 1986.

M. Fukuoka. *The Natural Way of Farming: The Theory and Practice of Green Philosophy*. New York: Japan Publications, Inc.. 1985.

E. Highbee. *Farms and Farmers in an Urban Age*. New York: The Twentieth Century Fund. 1963.

A. Howard. *An Agricultural Testament*. New York: Oxford University Press, 1943.

W. Jackson. *Altars of Unhewn Stone: Science and Earth*. San Francisco: North Point Press. 1987.

M. Kramer. *Three Farms*. Boston: Little Brown. 1977.

N.H. Lampkin and S. Padel, editors. *The Economics of Organic Farming: An International Perspective*. Wallingford, U.K.: CAB International.

F.M. Lappe, and J. Collins. *Food First. Beyond the Myth of Scarcity*. Boston: Houghton Mifflin. 1977.

R. Manning. *Grassland: The History, Biology and Promise of the American Prairie*. New York: Viking. 1995.

A.N. Martin. *Food Pets Die For: Shocking Facts About Pet Food*. Troutdale, Oregon: NewSage Press, 1997.

L. Marx. *The Machine in the Garden*. New York: Oxford University Press. 1964.

J.A. Montmarquet. *The Idea of Agrarianism*. Moscow: University of Idaho Press, 1989.

National Research Council. *Alternative Agriculture*. Washington, DC: Academy Press. 1989.

J. Paddock, N. Paddock, and C. Bly. *Soil and Survival. Land Stewardship and the Future of American Agriculture*. San Francisco: Sierra Club Books. 1986.

R.P. Poincelot. *Toward a More Sustainable Agriculture*. Westport, Connecticut: AVI Publishing. 1986.

J.R. Smith. *Tree Crops: A Permanent Agriculture*. Washington, DC: Island Press. 1950.

J. Solkoff. *The Politics of Food*. San Francisco: Sierra Club Books. 1985.

M. Strange. *Family Farming: A New Economic Vision*. Lincoln: University Nebraska Press. 1988.

J. Tivy. *Agricultural Ecology*. New York: John Wiley. 1990.

United Nations Development Programme. *Urban Agriculture: Food, Jobs and Sustainable Cities*. New York: UNDP. 1996.

GLOSSARY

Aflatoxin: a group of poisonous substances produced by a fungus (Aspergillus) on moldy foods.

Anabolic steroids: a class of hormones that stimulate metabolism.

Animal tankage: rendered remains of animals.

Avoparcine: one of a group of antibiotics used to control intestinal infections.

Bioethics: ethical principles relating to our treatment of the environment and all life.

Campylobacter: a class of intestinal bacteria.

Chlordane: highly toxic, chlorinated pesticide.

Clenbuterol: a drug that acts like an anabolic steroid.

Creutzfeld-Jakob disease: chronic, fatal degenerative brain disease in humans.

DDT: dichlorodiphenyltrichloroethane, a very toxic pesticide that persists in environment.

Dioxin: a poisonous class of industrial chemical pollutants with many toxic properties, notably causing hormonal (endocrine) disruptions.

E. coli: a common class of intestinal bacteria, most harmless.

EPA: United States Environmental Protection Agency.

Estrogen-mimicking chemicals: substances that act like natural hormones but disrupt normal functions.

EEC: The European Economic Community, a political body of the European Union.

FDA: United States federal government's Food and Drug Administration.

Free radicals: oxygen molecules that are natural byproducts of body metabolism that cause cell damage. The more food eaten, the more free radicals produced.

FSIS: United States Department of Agriculture's Food Safety Inspection Service.

GATT: the General Agreement on Trade and Tariffs, an international business convention.

GBS (Guillain-Barré syndrome): a progressive degenerative neurological disease.

Genistein: a highly beneficial hormone-like substance in soybeans.

HACCUP (or HASSUP): acronym for the FSIS new food safety protocol of hazard analysis at critical control points in meat processing.

Irradiation: exposure of various food products to atomic bombardment by radioactive materials like radium.

Lysteria moncytogenes: a class of intestinal bacteria.

Mad cow disease: a degenerative brain disease termed bovine spongiform encephalopathy (BSE).

Metabolites: breakdown products of cellular and digestive processes.

Monocropping: growing single crops without proper rotations to rest and enrich soils.

Nitrofurans: drugs used to treat bacterial infections.

Nutriceuticals: plant chemicals (phytochemicals) beneficial to human health.

Offal: entrails and other discarded and condemned parts of slaughtered animals.

Organochlorines: a group of highly toxic, chlorine-based pesticides.

PCBs: polychlorinated biphenyls used in industrial processes and discharged (with dioxins) from incinerators.

Phytochemicals: see Nutriceuticals.

Piscitarian: neologism for those who eat no animal products except fish.

Premarin: brand name for estrogen-replacement medication derived from pregnant mare's urine.

Prion: protein-based infectious particles that can cause degenerative brain disease in humans and other animals.

Rendering: process of disposing of offal and dead animals using heat, chemicals and mechanical maceration.

Ruminants: animals with four stomachs enabling them to digest plant cellulose.

Salmonella: a class of intestinal bacteria that are a common cause of food poisoning.

SARE/Sustainable Agriculture Research and Education: program of the U.S. Department of Agriculture.

SHBG: a blood protein (globulin) that helps regulate levels of circulating sex hormones.

Transgenic: animals (and plants) that carry alien genes from other species as a result of being genetically engineered.

Trenbolon acetate: one of several synthetic sex hormone implants that increase animals' growth and metabolism: less fat and more muscle.

USDA: United States Department of Agriculture, a federal agency.

Vegan: one who eats no animal product, dairy, eggs, meat, or fish.

Vegetarian: one who does not eat meat or fish, but maybe eggs and dairy products.

WTO: World Trade Organization, established on the foundation of the GATT.

Zeranol: a synthetic sex hormone implant used to stimulate growth and reduce fat in cattle raised for meat.

ENDNOTES

Chapter One: Why Eat With Conscience?

1.George Eisman, with Anne Green, and Matt Ball. *The Most Noble Diet: Food Selection and Ethics*. New York: Diet Ethics. 1994.

Chapter Two: Factory Farming: A Holocaust in the Animal Kingdom

1. According to a 1986 report by the Office of Technology Assessment, animal disease cost U.S. agriculture $17 billion annually. (*Feedstuffs*, March 14, 1994).

2. John Robbins. *Diet for a New America*. Walpole, New Hampshire: Stillpoint Publishing. 1987. pp. 56, 57; and Jim Mason. "The incredible egg story." *Vegetarian Times*. Oak Park, Illinois. 101: 225-26. January 1986; and David C. Coats, *Old MacDonald's Factory Farm, The Myth of the Traditional Farm and the Shocking Truth About Animal Suffering in Today's Agribusiness*. New York: Continuum Publishers, Inc. 1980. p. 85.

3. *Diet for a New America*. pp. 59-60.

4. Ibid. pp. 84, 88, 89; and Jim Mason and Peter Singer. *Animal Factories*. New York: Crown Publishers, Inc. 1980. pp. 22-24.

5. R. Jensen, et al. "Abomasal erosion in feedlot cattle. *American Journal of Veterinary Research* 53:110-15. 1992.

6. T. Grandin, editor. *Livestock Handling and Transportation*. Wallingford, Oxford: CAB International. 1993.

7. *Feedstuffs*. p. 59. May 2, 1994.

8. United States Department of Agriculture. *Agricultural Research*. Washington, DC: USDA. 39:7-8. 1991.

9. *Lancaster Farming*. October 27, 1990.

10. According to the *FAO Production Yearbook 1990*. (Rome, 1991), UN Food and Agriculture Organization, some 1,764 pounds of grains are used to feed livestock in the U.S. to meet the annual per capita average consumption of 93 pounds beef, 44 pounds pork, 97 pounds poultry, 624 pounds dairy products, and 35 pounds of eggs.

11. National Research Council. *Alternative Agriculture*. Washington, DC: National Academy Press. 1989.

12. United States Department of Agriculture. *National Swine Survey*. Washington, DC: USDA. 1992.

13. United States Department of Agriculture. *Agricultural Research*. Washington, DC: USDA. p. 23. February 1993.

14. The FDA's clear support of drug company interests and limited authority in protecting consumer interests is exemplified by the fact that close to 90 percent of all food animal drugs are approved for OTC (over the counter) sales to farmers and ranchers (see *DVM Magazine*, p. 32. January 1993). Most drugs should be available only through a veterinarian whose responsibility and professional training ensures their safe and effective use.

15. H.C. New. "The crisis in antibiotic resistance." *Science*. 257:1064-78. 1992; see also, M.L. Cohen. "Epidemiology of drug resistance: implications for a post-antimicrobial era. *Science*. 257:1050-5. 1991; see also, Office of Technology Assessment. *Impact of Antibiotic Resistant Bacteria*. Washington, DC: U.S. Government Printing Office. 1995.

16. B. Wuethrich. "Migrating genes could spread resistance." *New Scientist*. p. 9. October 15, 1994.

17. See: "Watch out for killer algae." *E Magazine*. March/April. pp. 15-18. 1996.

18. Dr. Gary Cromwell, University of Kentucky livestock management specialist, cited in *Feedstuffs*. July 25, 1994.

19. L.A. Kerr, et al. "Chronic copper poisoning in sheep grazing pastures fertilized with swine manure." *Journal of the American Veterinary Medical Association*. 198:99-101. 1991.

20. S.W. Casteel, et al. "Selenium toxicosis in swine." *Journal of the American Veterinary Medical Association*. 186:1084-85. 1985.

21. L.H. Harrison, et al. "Paralysis in swine due to focal symmetrical poliomalacia; possible selenium toxicosis." *Veterinary Pathology*. 20:265-73. 1983.

22. T.M. Wilson, et al. "Selenium toxicity and porcine focal symmetrical poliomyelomalacia: description of a field outbreak and experimental reproduction." *Canadian Journal of Comparative Medicine*. 47:412-21. 1983.

23. J. Hill, et al. "An episode of acute selenium toxicity in a commercial piggery." *Australian Veterinary Journal*. 62:207-9. 1985.

24. P.H. Anderson, et al. "Suspected selenium poisoning in lambs." *Veterinary Record*. 116:647. 1985.

25. H.D. Stowe, et al. "Selenium toxicosis in feeder pigs." *Journal of American Veterinary Medical Association*. 201:292-95. 1992.

26. *American Journal of Alternative Agriculture*. 1-2, 63-68. 1992.

27. For a comprehensive review of this fascinating and important aspect of the human-animal bond, see, P.H. Hemsworth, et al. "The human-animal relationship in agriculture and its consequences for the animal." *Animal Welfare*. Universities Federation for Welfare. 2:33-51. 1993.

28. For details, see: M.F. Seabrook. "The effect of production systems on the behavior and attitudes of stockpersons." *Biological Basis of Sustainable Animal Production*. Proceedings of 4th Zodiac Symposium. Waneningen, The Netherlands: EAAP Publication. 67: 252-8. 1994.

29. J. Fahy. "All pain, no gain." *Southern Exposure*. 17:2. 1989; and "Fishy business." *Southern Exposure*. 19:3. 1991; and D. Cecelski and M.L. Kerr. "Hog wild." *Southern Exposure*. 20:3. 1992.

30. K.J. Donham and K.M. Thu. "Relationships of agricultural and economic policy to the health of farm families, livestock, and the environment." *Journal of American Veterinary Medical Association*. 202:1084-91. April 1, 1993.

31. For a detailed investigation of BSE, see Richard Rhoades, *Deadly Feasts: Tracking the Secrets of a Terrifying New Plague*. New York: Simon and Schuster. 1997.

32. Ann N. Martin. *Food Pets Die For: Shocking Facts About Pet Food*. Troutdale, Oregon: NewSage Press. 1997.

33. "Feed, animal flatulence and atmosphere." *Washington Post*. p. A6. December 12, 1988.

34. F.M. Byers and N.D. Turner. "The role of methane from beef cattle in global warming." *Beef Cattle Research in Texas*. College Station, Texas: Texas Agricultural Experiment Station. PR-4838. pp. 69-74. June 1991..

35. A. Mosler, et al. "Methane and nitrous oxide fluxes in native, fertilized and cultivated grasslands." *Nature*. 350:330-2. 1991.

36. *Progressive Farmer*. June/July 1997.

Chapter Three: The Rotten Roots of Agribusiness

1. A critical need for health insurance and pensions is cause for many farmers to seek off-farm employment. According to agricultural economist, Dr. David Kohl, less than half of America's two million farms have profit potential, averaging $3 in debt for every $1 of net income. Eighty percent of all farm income is earned by just 20 percent of the farms, and only one in five farms earns more than a 10 percent return on profits. (*Feedstuffs*, February 22, 1993.)

2. United States Department of Agriculture. "The US Farming Sector Entering the 1990s: Twelfth Annual Report on the Status of Family Farms." *Agriculture Information Bulletin 587*. Washington, DC: USDA. June 1990; and United States Department of Agriculture. "Financial Characteristics of US Farms." Washington, DC: USDA. January 1, 1989.

3. Roger Runningen. "USDA's Glickman endorses review of meatpacker concentration." *Bloomberg* wire story. Oct. 18, 1995; and "AG economist's moderate farm shakeout under farm bill." *Financial World News* wire story. March 7, 1996.

4. M. Crouch in: *The Agriculture Bioethics Forum*. Ames, Iowa: Iowa State University. 4:5-6. 1992.

5. A.V. Krebs. *The Corporate Reapers: The Book of Agribusiness*. Washington, DC: Essential Books. 1992.

Endnotes

6. For an excellent review and documentation, see: W.C. Lowdermilk. *Conquest of the Land Through 7000 Years.* Agricultural Information Bulletin 99. Washington DC: United States Department of Agriculture, Soil Conservation Service. 1975.

7. *Our Food Our World: Realities of an Animal-Based Diet.* Santa Cruz, California: EarthSave Foundation. p. 9. March, 1992.

8. For further documentation, see: R. Repetto and S.S. Baliga. *Pesticides and the Immune System: The Public Health Risks.* Baltimore, Maryland: World Resources Institute. 1996; T. Colburn, D. Dumanoski, and J.P. Myers. *Our Stolen Future: Are We Threatening Our Fertility, Intelligence and Survival? A Scientific Detective Story.* New York: Dutton. 1996; L.M. Gibbs. *Dying from Dioxin: A Citizen's Guide to Reclaiming Our Health and Rebuilding Democracy.* Boston, Massachusetts: South End Press. 1995; and *Fertility on the Brink.* Washington, DC: National Wildlife Federation. 1994.

9. National Academy of Sciences. *Pesticides in the Diets of Infants and Children.* Washington DC: National Academy of Sciences Press. 1993.

10. Philip J. Landrigna, pediatrician, chair of the National Academy of Sciences Committee. *Washington Post.* June 28, 1993.

11. National Academy of Sciences. *Toxicity Testing: Strategies to Determine Needs and Priorities.* Washington, DC: National Academy of Sciences Press. 1984.

12. *Successful Farming.* p. 24. March 1994.

13. "Farm cancer risk elevated." *Washington Post.* September 23, 1992.

14. D. Pimental. *Handbook on Pest Management in Agriculture.* Boca Raton: Florida: CRC Press. 1991.

15. National Research Council. *Regulating Pesticides in Food: The Delaney Paradox.* Washington, DC: National Academy Press. 1987.

16. John Robbins. *Diet for a New America.* Walpole, New Hampshire: Stillpoint Publishing. 1987. p. 343.

17. Ibid. pp. 314-316; Jeremy Rifkin. *Beyond Beef: The Rise and Fall of the Cattle Culture.* New York: Penguin. pp. 12-13; and "Is our fish fit to eat?" *Consumer Reports.* Yonkers, NY: Consumers Union. 57:2:112,114. February 1992; *EarthSave.* p. 7. Spring 1996.

18. D. Pimental. *Handbook on Pest Management in Agriculture.* Boca Raton, Florida: CRC Press. 1991; also, "Environmental and economic costs of pesticide use." *BioScience.* 42: 750-60. 1992.

19. World Health Organization. *Public Health Impact of Pesticides Used in Agriculture.* Geneva, Switzerland: World Health Organization Press. 1990.

20. *What Americans Think About Agrichemicals.* Washington, DC: Public Voice for Food and Health Policy. 1993.

21. "Tap water blues." Washington, DC: Environmental Working Group. October 1994.

22. *Food Chemical News.* p. 33. January 9, 1995.

23. Craig Cramer, et al. *Controlling Weeds with Fewer Chemicals: How to Cut Herbicide Costs and Protect the Environment.* Emmaus, Pennsylvania: Rodale Press. 1994.

24. Arnold Schecter, et al, at State University of New York (Syracuse), Department of Preventive Medicine. *Food Chemical News.* p. 25. January 23, 1995.

25. "Is your food safe?" "48 Hours." CBS-TV. February 9, 1994.

26. Resenfeld, et al. *A Menu for Food Safety Failures: What the Bush Administration is Serving Consumers.* Washington, DC: Public Voice for Food and Health Policy. p. 5. June 1992; and Nora Macaluso. "USDA's new poultry rules won't be tough enough, group says." *Bloomberg* wire story. March 13, 1996; and Testimony from Hearing of the Committee on Labor and Human Resources, U.S. Senate on *Poultry Safety; Consumers at Risk.* p. 236. June 28, 1991.

27. Family Food Protection Act of 1995 (Section 515); "House panel blocks new meat inspection rules in farm money bill." Roger Runningen at the USDA. *Bloomberg* wire story. June 27, 1995.

28. University of Kentucky, reported in the *Food Chemical News.* p. 48. December 5, 1994.

29. *Food Chemical News.* p. 26. May 9, 1994.

30. "Guaranteed safe meat?" *Journal of the American Veterinary Medical Association.* 206:432-33. 1995.

31. Further insights into the abuse of the public land grazing subsidies by ranchers were provided by John Horning, Director, Headwaters Campaign, Forest Guardians, Santa Fe, New Mexico, in his letter to the *Washington Post.* January 31, 1995.

32. "Angry ranchers across the west see grounds for an insurrection." *Washington Post.* February 21, 1995.

33. According to Edward R. Madican, former Secretary of Agriculture in testimony before the Senate Subcommittee on Agriculture, Rural Development, and Related Agencies. February 25, 1992.

34. E. Goldsmith and N. Hildyard, editors. *The Earth Report 2: Monitoring the Battle for the Environment.* London: Mitchell Beazley. p. 167. 1990.

35. For a detailed discussion of water shortage in the U.S. and the politics of agricultural irrigation, see: M. Reissner, *Cadillac Desert: The Amerian West and Its Disappearing Water.* London: Seeker and Warburg. 1990.

36. Masanobu Fukuoka. *The Natural Way of Farming.* New York: Japan Publications, Inc. 1985.

37. Todd Oppenheimer. "The rancher subsidy." *Atlantic Monthly.* pp. 26-38. January 1996.

38. B. Rensberger. "Alarm for nature's bounty." *Washington Post.* p. A3. April 6. 1992; and "Many farm animal breeds risk extinction, UN experts say." *New York Times International.* December 7, 1995.

39. *Washington Post.* May 16, 1993.

40. Ibid.

41. Ibid.

Chapter Four: Genetic Engineering and Biomedical Research

1. M.W. Fox. *Super pigs and Wonder Corn: The Brave New World of Biotechnology and Where It All May Lead.* New York: Lyons and Burford. 1992.

2. *The Gene Exchange.* December 1991.

3. United States Department of Agriculture. *Agriculture Fact Book.* Washington, DC: USDA. p. 188. 1966

4. Lisa Levin. "Farm animals research warrants close attention." *W.A.R.D. S.* Vienna, Virginia. p2. Spring 1995.

5. Paula Maas, Susan E. Brown, and Nancy Bruning. *The MEND Clinic Guide to Natural Medicine for Menopause and Beyond.* New York: Dell Publishing. 1997. p. 69.

6. T.J. Hoban and P.A. Kendall, USDA Extension Service. *Consumer Attitudes About the Use of Biotechnology in Agriculture and Food Production.* July 1992.

7. *Safe Food News.* Winter 1995; and Bio/Technology/Diversity Week. March 14, 1995.

8. *Wisconsin Farmers Union News* release. March 14, 1995.

9. S.S. Epstein. "Unlabeled milk from cows treated with biosynthetic growth hormones: a case of regulatory abdication." *International Journal of Health Services.* 26:173:85. 1996.

Chapter Five: A Sea of Troubled Waters: Factory Fishing and Aquaculture

1. A. Swardson. "Net losses: fishing decimating oceans' 'unlimited bounty.'" *Washington Post.* p. 1, A28-29. August 14, 1994.

2. Ibid.

3. Carl Safina. "The worlds' imperiled fish." *Scientific American.* pp. 46-33. 1995.

4. For further documentation see: P. Lymbery, *The Welfare of Farmed Fish.* Hants, England: Compassion in World Farming. 1992; and G.K. Iwama, "Interactions between aquaculture and the environment." *Critical Reviews in Environmental Control.* 21:177-216. 1991.

Endnotes

5. F.P. Myers. *Journal of Animal Science*. 69:4201-8. 1991.

6. *Food Chemical News*. p. 36. October 10, 1994.

7. H. Kane. "Growing fish in fields." *World Watch Institute*. 6:20-7. 1993.

8. M. Fishchetti. "A feast of gene-splicing down on the fish farm." *Science*. 253:512-3. 1991.

9. *Washington Post*. p. A3. December 1, 1996.

10. T. Colburn, D. Dumanoski, and J.P. Myers. *Our Stolen Future: Are We Threatening Our Fertility, Intelligence and Survival? A Scientific Detective Story*. New York: Dutton. 1996.

11. Marion Burros. "Eating well: a start for regulating U.S. seafood." *New York Times*. p. C4. November 29, 1995.

Chapter Six: Beware: You Are What You Eat

1. *New York Times*. March 30, 1993.

2. R. J. Kuezmarski, et al. "Increasing prevalence of overweight among U.S. adults." *Journal of the American Medical Association*. National Center for Health Statistics. 272:205-11. 1994.

3. NBC-TV News report. July 19, 1994.

4. Paul E. Waggoner. *How Much Land Can Ten Billion People Spare for Nature?* Ames, Iowa: Council for Agricultural Science and Technology. 1994.

5. *Milwaukie Journal Sentinel*. pp. 1, 13. June 11, 1996.

6. The Humane Farming Association press release. January 21, 1997.

7. The Department of Justice issued a news summary of its investigation, November 1996. The department is negotiating with the Dutch government for the extradition of Gerard Hoogendijk, the principal supplier of black market drugs from The Netherlands to stand trial in the U.S. A federal grand jury in Milwaukee, Wisconsin returned an indictment against Travis Calf Milk, Inc., a Wisconsin-based veal formula company and its president Gerald R. Travis for his purchase of one hundred fifty thousand pounds of tainted veal feed supplements from Vitek. He pleaded guilty to one count of criminal conspiracy to defraud the U.S. government. The grand jury also indicted VIV, Inc. (aka Hying America), one of the largest veal factory farms, and its operators Hennie and Jan Van Den Hengel for their roles in smuggling unapproved drugs into the United States for use in veal feed. Charges were also filed against Wisconsin-based Provimi Veal Corporation for violating food and drug laws. In addition to clenbuterol, other unapproved drugs involved in this investigation include the antibiotic avoparcine and potentially carcinogenic nitrofurans. Source: Gail Eisnitz, "More convictions of veal industry leaders in clenbuterol case." *Humane Farming Association's Special Report*. August 1997.

8. 4-D meat is the *official* term given to the meat derived from animals that are diseased, debilitated, dying, or dead on arrival at the slaughterhouse.

9. L.P. Williams, Jr. *Journal of the American Veterinary Medical Association*. 201:12-3. 1992.

10. P. Giem, et al. *Adventist Health Study: Neuroepidemiology*. 12:28-36. 1993.

11. M.E. Szczawinska, D.W. Thayer, and J.G. Phillips. "Fate of irradiated *Salmonella* in irradiated mechanically deboned chicken meat." *International Journal of Food Medicine*. 14:313-24. 1991.

12. *FDA Strategy Needed to Address Animal Drug Residues In Milk*. Gaithersburg, Maryland: General Accounting Office. GAO/RCED: 92-209. 1994.

13. W.J. Cole, et al. "Response of dairy cows to high doses of a sustained-release bovine somatotropin administered during two lactations." *Journal of Dairy Science*. 75:111-23. 1991.

14. M.B. Zemel. "Calcium utilization: effects of varying level and source of dietary protein." *American Journal of Clinical Nutrition*. 48:880-3. 1988.

15. P.S. Clyne and A. Kulczyck. "Human breast milk contains bovine lgc. relationship to infant colic." *Pediatrics*. 87:439-4. 1991.

16. R.R.A. Coombs and S.T. Holgate. "Allergy and cot death: with special focus on allergic sensitivity to cow's milk and anaphylaxis." *Clinical and Experimental Allergy*. 20:3509-66. 1990.

17. J. Rennie. "Formula for diabetes?" *Scientific American*. pp. 24-25. October 1992.

18. J. Karjalaainen, J.M. Martin, M. Knip, et al. "A bovine albumin peptide as a possible trigger of insulin-dependent diabetes mellitus." *New England Journal of Medicine*. 327:302-7. 1991.

19. F.W. Scott. "Cow milk and insulin-dependent diabetes mellitus: is there a relationship?" *American Journal of Clinical Nutrition*. 51:489-91. 1990.

20. American Academy of Pediatrics, Committee on Nutrition. "The use of whole cow's milk in infancy." *Pediatrics*. 89-1105-9. 1992.

21. E.E. Ziegler, S.J. Fomon, S.E. Nelson, et al. "Cow milk feeding in infancy: further observations on blood loss from gastrointestinal tract." *Journal of Pediatrics*. 116:11-8. 1993.

22. D. Olwens, et al. "Circulating testosterone levels and aggression in adolescent males: a causal analysis." *Psychosomatic Medicine*. 50:261-272. 1988.

23. H. Adlercreutz. "Western diet and western diseases: some hormonal and biochemical mechanisms and associations." *Scandinavian Journal of Clinical and Laboratory Investigation*. 50 Suppl. 201:3-23. 1990.

24. A. Belanger, A. Locong, C. Noel, et al. "Influence on diet on plasma steroid and sex hormone binding globulin levels in adult men." *Journal Steroid Biochemistry*. 32:829-33. 1989.

25. Neal Barnard. *Eat Right, Live Longer*. New York: Crown Books. 1993.

26. A. Gray, D.N. Jackson, J.B. McKinlay. "The relation between dominance, anger, and hormones in normally aging men: results from the Massachusetts male aging study." *Psychosomatic Medicine*. 53:375-85. 1991.

27. F.G.R. Fowkes, et al. "Serum cholesterol, triglycerides and aggression in the general population." *The Lancet*. 3240: 1995-98. 1992.

Chapter Seven: Power of the Plate: Eating for a Greener World

1. Linda Rosenweig. *New Vegetarian Cuisine*. Emmaus, Pennsylvania: Rodale Press. 1994.

2. For further discussion, see R.W. Lacey, "Disease Transfer," Chapter 21, *Farm Animals and the Environment*. C. Philips and D. Piggins, editors. London: C.A.B. International. 1993.

3. "More evidence found on diet's role in cancer." *Washington Post*. October 7, 1992.

4. "Death rate cut in half for vegetarians, German study finds." *Food Chemical News*. p. 10. September 21, 1992.

5. L.E. Aspnes, et al. "Caloric restriction reduces fiber loss and mitochondrial abnormalities in aged rat muscle." *Journal of the Federation of American Societies for Experimental Biology* 11: 573:581. 1997.

6. W.C. Willett. "Diet and health: what should we eat?" *Science*. 224:532-7. 1994.

7. "Diet and chronic degenerative diseases: perspectives from China." *American Journal of Clinical Nutrition*. Suppl: 59: 1153S-61S. 1994; and see also, N.J. Temple and Densi P. Burkitt, editors. *Western Diseases, Their Dietary Prevention and Reversibility*. Totowa, New Jersey: Humana Press. 1994.

8. Neal Barnard. *Food for Life*. New York: Crown Publishers. 1993.

9. M. Fukuoka. *The Natural Way of Farming*. New York: Japan Publications. 1985.

10. B.H. Arjmandi, et al. "Dietary soybean protein prevents bone loss in an ovariectomized rat model of osteoporosis." *Journal of Nutrition*. 126:161-167. 1996.

11. *New Scientist*. pp. 14-15. July 9, 1994.

12. "Huge study of diet indicts fat and meat." *New York Times*. May 8, 1990.

Endnotes

13. Hans-Michael Dosch, et al. *New England Journal of Medicine.* July 30, 1992.

14. M. Thorogood, J. Mann, P. Appleby, K. McPherson. "Risk of death from cancer and ischaemic heart disease in meat and non-meat eater." *British Medical Journal.* 308:1167(4). 1994.

15. T. Sanders and S. Reddy. "Vegetarian diets and children." *American Journal of Clinical Nutrition.* 59 Suppl:12176S-81S. 1994.

16. Linda Rosenweig. *New Vegetarian Cuisine.* Emmaus, Pennsylvania: Rodale Press. 1994.

Chapter Eight: Stopping the Wasteland

1. World Resources Institute, Washington, DC, in collaboration with the United Nations Environmental Program. 1992.

2. J.P. Reganold, et al. "Soil quality and financial performance of biodynamic and conventional farms in New Zealand." *Science.* 260:344-9. 1993; see also: V. Klinkenborg. "A farming revolution. "*National Geographic.* 188:60-89. December 1995.

3. D. Pimental. "Environmental and social implications of waste in U.S. agriculture and food sectors." *Journal of Agricultural Ethics.* 3:1-12. 1990.

4. H. Waller. *Earth Island Journal.* pp. 32-33. Spring 1990.

5. For more information see: A. Lee, *Chicken Tractor: The Gardener's Guide to Happy Hens and Healthy Soil.* Columbus, North Carolina: Good Earth Publications. 1994; see also: K. Thear. *Free Range Poultry.* Ipswich, United Kingdom: Farming Press. 1990.

6. J. Salatin. *Pastured Poultry Profits.* Swoope, Virginia: Polyface, Inc. 1994.

7. M. Honeyman. "Sustainable swine production." *Farming Systems for Iowa: Seeking Alternatives.* Conference proceedings. Iowa State University, Ames, Iowa: Leopold Center for Sustainable Agriculture. 1990.

8. For more information see: K. Thornton, *Outdoor Pig Production.* Ipswich, United Kingdom: Farming Press. 1990.

9. C. Cramer. "Pastures beat BGH: farmers, consumers and rural communities all win with rotational grazing, says this new study." *The New Farm.* July/August 1991.

10. W.C. Liebhardt, editor. *The Dairy Debate, Consequences of Bovine Growth Hormone and Rotational Grazing Technologies.* Davis, California: University of California Press. 1993.

11. M.K. Gandhi. *My Socialism.* Ahmedabad: Navajivan Publishing House. 1959. pp. 34-35.

12. *Which Row to Hoe? A Regional Perspective on Alternative Directions in Commercial Agriculture.* St. Paul, Minnesota: Northwest Area Foundation. May 1992; see also: S. Schmickle. "Sustainable farming viable study suggest." *Minnesota Star Tribune.* June 20, 1992.

13. *Detroit News.* October 5, 1992.

14. Ontario Department of Agriculture. *Duck and Goose Raising.* No. 532. 1992.

15. *New Scientist.* 18. April 16, 1994.

Chapter Nine: Change of Conscience: Actions and Solutions

1. Chefs Collaborative 2000, 25 First Street, Cambridge, Massachusetts 02141. Reprinted by permission.

INDEX

Index

Index

Nippon Meat Packers, 55
nitrofurans, 110
nitrous oxide, 46
non-Hodgkins lymphoma, 62
North America, fish as source of protein in, 106
North Carolina,
  abuses in, 42
  manure spills in, 36
Northwest Area Foundation (NAF), 149, 151
Norway, 106, 144
Novartis, 81
nutriceuticals, 137

O
obesity, 117
Ogallala Aquifer, 75
Oklahoma, 42
omega-3 fatty acids, 113
organic,
  farming, 102, 144-146
  foods, 40
  labeling, 102
Organic Food Production Act 1990, 82, 144
organoleptic inspection, 66-67
Oscar Mayer Foods, 55
osteoporosis,
  cause of, 116
  hens with, 33
  preventing, 137
overfishing, 105-108
overgrazing, 65, 143, 150
oxytetracycline, 110
oysters, 112

P
Pacific salmon, 109
packing plant. See slaughterhouse
pale-soft-exudative (PSE), 29, 124
PCBs, 60-62, 112
pelicans, 108
penguins, 108
personality changes, 41-42, 123-125
pest control methods, 63, 151, 152
pesticides, 36, 44, 60-62, 86, 109, 112
petrels, 108
pet food, 43, 45, 65, 107, 120, 163
pets, 66, 163
Pfiesteria piscidia, 36
"pharming", 92, 95
phosphates, 16, 37, 39
phytochemicals, 137
pigs,
  abuses to, 27-30, 33, 88
  antibiotics in feed, 35
  piglets, 27, 33
Pillsbury, 77
Pimental, David, 60, 63
piscitarian, 130
pneumonia in hogs and humans, 32
polar bear, 107
polyunsaturated fatty acids, 132
Pork Producers Congress, 30
potassium permanganate, 110
poultry,
  abuse to, 16, 26
  business dangerous, 57
  production-related diseases to, 26, 33-34
"power of the plate," 127
Premium Standard Farms, 48
Premarin, 89, 90
Prestige Farms, 48
price,
  fixing, 54-59, 74, 78-79
  supports, 78, 166
Prima Meat Packers, 55
prion, 44, 168
Produce for Better Health Foundation, 132
production unit, animal considered as, 14, 25-31
prostate cancer, 123
Provimi Veal Corporation, 118
Public Voice for Food and Health Policy, 64
puffins, 108
Pure Food Campaign, 80

Q
quinolones, 110

R
Rainforest Action Network, 156
ranch
  See also overgrazing
  demise of, 14, 22
  hands, 41
rangeland and methane gas, 46, 151
ranchers' rights, 71
rBGH, See recombinant bovine growth hormone
  (rBGH)
Reagan administration, 51
rebreeding difficulties in cows, 32
recombinant bovine growth hormone (rBGH), 96-101,
  121-123
Reddy, S., 138
rendering plants, 43, 45, 65
Rhoades, Richard, 18
RJR Nabisco, 54
Royal Agricultural Society of the United Kingdom, 38
Russia, 78

S
Sadia Group, 55
Salatin, Joel, 147
salmon,
  See also fish
  antifreeze genes in, 85
  eating, 112
  farmers, 108, 109
Salmonella, 34, 67, 68, 69, 120, 121
Sanders, T., 138
San Joaquin Valley, 75
Sara Lee, 55
scrapie, 88, 168
Seaboard Corporation, 48
Seabrook, M.F., 41-42
seafood
  See also fish
  safety of eating, 112, 131
sea lice, 109
seals, 108
sea trout, 109
selenium, 39-40
SHBG, 123
sheep,
  See also BSE; cloning; scrapie
  grazing, 150
  in biomedical research, 88, 94-96
shrimp, 108, 109-112
Shumway, John, 98
Simazine, 64
skin, animal, products, 164
slaughterhouse,
  numbers of animals killed in, 13
  psychological effects on workers, 40-43
  stress of animals in, 40-43, 69, 124
  transport to, 29-30, 45
Smithfield Foods, 48
soy products, 73, 136, 137, 150
sperm count, 62
starvation of cattle, 71
stress in animals,
  during confinement, 41
  during transport, 29-30
subsidies, 24, 69-75, 149-151, 166
subsidized public lands, 69-73
Sunniest Growers, 77
sustainable agriculture, 147-153
Sustainable Agriculture Research and Education
  (SARE), 72, 81
Swardson, Anne, 106, 108
Sweden, 144
Switzerland, 144
synergism, 61

T
tankage, animal, 43-44
  See also BSE
taxpayers' expense, 17, 24, 36, 48, 70, 77-79
Taylor, Michael, 101
Texas, 75, 80
Texas Commission of Agriculture, 60
Thailand, 44
tilapia, 109, 112
Toiyabe National Forest, 71
topsoil erosion, 16, 19, 25, 72, 143
transgenic,
  See also cloning

farm animals, 93-94
foods, 87
transportation, cost of, 29-30, 58
trash fish, 107
Tyson Foods, 55, 77, 78

U
Unilever, 54
union busting, 57
Union International, 55
United Kingdom, 44, 45, 62, 83
United Nations Food and Agriculture Organization
  (FAO), 105, 106, 108
United States Department of Agriculture (USDA),
  and branding policy, 29
  and genetically engineered crops, 86
  and pesticide policy, 61
  Animal and Plant Health Inspection Service,
    See Animal and Plant Health Inspection Service
    (APHIS)
  budget, 82
  Economic Research Service Food Safety Branch, 34
  Extension Service, 91
  Food Guide Pyramid, 134
  inspection, 66-67
  National Agricultural Statistics Services, 115
United States Forest Service, 70-71
USDA, See United States Department of Agriculture
United States Oceanic and Atmospheric
  Administration, 107

V
Van Noppen, Karl, 119
veal,
  calves, 16, 24, 25
  companies, investigation of, 118-119
  milk-fed, 25
vegan, 130
vegetarianism, 127, 132, 139
Vitek Supply Corporation, 119
violence, See food and emotions
Vogel, Lyle P., 69

W
Waggoner, Paul E., 118, 129
walrus, 107
waste, See manure
water,
  cost for animal production, 23
  irrigation, See irrigation
  hazards to health, 64-66
  pollution of, 36-37
weed control using animals, 150-151
wetlands, 74, 82
Weindruch, Richard, 132
whales, 107-108
Williams, Leslie P., 120
Willett, Walter C., 133
Wilmut, Ian, 94
Wisconsin Farmers Union, 98
Wisconsin Medical School, 117
Welch's, 77
World Trade Organization (WTO), 78, 79
World War II nerve gas, 52
Wyeth-Ayerst Laboratories, 88

Z
Zenchiku Co., 55
zinc, 39-40, 131, 139

About the Author

Michael W. Fox joined The Humane Society of the United States (The HSUS) in Washington, D.C., in 1976. Over the years he has worked extensively in animal reform. He currently serves as Vice President of Bioethics for Humane Society International and Senior Advisor to the President for The HSUS. In addition, he is on the Board of Directors for the Center of Respect of Life and Environment, an affiliate of The HSUS.

Michael Fox has also developed several technical research programs that applied scientific methods to the investigation of the many uses of animals, notably laboratory, companion, and farm animals. Fox has written extensively on many aspects of animals, and has more than forty books, some of which have received special recognition or science awards. Fox has a nationwide syndicated newspaper column, "Ask Your Animal Doctor." He is also a consulting veterinarian, and gives lectures, seminars and presentations both in the United States and abroad on a variety of topics related to animal welfare, behavior, conservation, and bioethics.

Dr. Fox has a veterinary degree from London's Royal Veterinary College, and a Ph.D. in medicine and a D.Sc. in ethology/animal behavior, both from London University, England. He is profiled in *Who's Who in America* and in *Who's Who in the World*.

Some Other Books by Dr. Michael W. Fox

♦ *The Boundless Circle* (1996) Quest Books, Wheaton, Illinois.

♦ *Agricide: The Hidden Farm and Food Crisis That Affects Us All* (reprint edition 1996) Krieger Publishing Co., Melbourne, Florida.

♦ *Super Pigs and Wonder Corn: The Brave New World of Biotechnology and Where It All Might Lead* (1992) Lyons & Burford, New York.

♦ *The Soul of The Wolf* (reprint edition 1992) Lyons & Burford, New York.

♦ *Inhumane Society: The American Way of Exploiting Animals* (1990) St. Martin's Press, New York.

♦ *The New Animal Doctor's Answer Book* (1989) Newmarket Press, New York.

♦ *Laboratory Animal Husbandry* (1986) State University of New York Press, Albany.

♦ *Between Animal and Man: The Key to the Kingdom.* (reprint edition 1986) Krieger Publishing Co., Melbourne, Florida.

♦ *Farm Animals: Husbandry, Behavior and Veterinary Practice* (1983) University Press, Baltimore, Maryland.

♦ *Returning to Eden: Animal Rights and Human Responsibility* (1980) Viking Press, New York.

Books by NewSage Press

Food Pets Die For: Shocking Facts About Pet Food
Ann N. Martin
Foreword by Dr. Michael W. Fox

The Wolf, the Woman, the Wilderness: A True Story of Returning Home
Teresa tsimmu Martino

Dancer on the Grass: True Stories of Horses and People
Teresa tsimmu Martino
(Available Spring 1998)

Animals as Teachers & Healers: True Stories & Reflections
Susan Chernak McElroy
(first published by NewSage, now available through Ballantine)

One Woman, One Vote: Rediscovering the Woman Suffrage Movement
edited by Marjorie Spruill Wheeler

Jailed for Freedom: American Women Win the Vote
Doris Stevens, edited by Carol O'Hare

Women & Work: In Their Own Words
edited by Maureen R. Michelson

Blue Moon Over Thurman Street
Ursula K. Le Guin
Photographs by Roger Dorband

When the Bough Breaks: Pregnancy & the Legacy of Addiction
Kira Corser & Frances Payne Adler

A Portrait of American Mothers & Daughters
Raisa Fastman

Organizing for Our Lives: New Voices from Rural Communities
Richard Steven Street & Samuel Orozco

Family Portraits in Changing Times
Helen Nestor

Stories of Adoption: Loss & Reunion
Eric Blau, M.D.

Common Heroes: Facing a Life Threatening Illness
Eric Blau, M.D.